LISTENING TO SCENT

by the same author

A Sensory Journey
Meditations on Scent for Wellbeing
Card set
ISBN 978 1 84819 153 2
eISBN 978 0 85701 175 6

Fragrance and Wellbeing
Plant Aromatics and Their Influence on the Psyche
ISBN 978 1 84819 090 0
eISBN 978 0 85701 073 5

Essential Oils
A Handbook for Aromatherapy Practice
2nd edition
ISBN 978 1 84819 089 4
eISBN 978 0 85701 072 8

LISTENING
TO SCENT

An Olfactory Journey with
Aromatic Plants and Their Extracts

JENNIFER PEACE RHIND

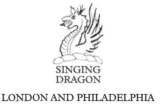

SINGING
DRAGON
LONDON AND PHILADELPHIA

First published in 2014
by Singing Dragon
an imprint of Jessica Kingsley Publishers
73 Collier Street
London N1 9BE, UK
and
400 Market Street, Suite 400
Philadelphia, PA 19106, USA

www.singingdragon.com

Library of Congress Cataloging in Publication Data
Rhind, Jennifer.
  Listening to scent : an olfactory journey with aromatic plants and their extracts / Jennifer Peace Rhind.
    pages cm
  Includes bibliographical references and index.
  ISBN 978-1-84819-125-9 (alk. paper)
  1. Odors--Psychological aspects. 2. Aromatic plants. 3. Essences and essential oils. 4. Aromatherapy.
  I. Title.
  RM666.A68R53 2014
  615.3'219--dc23
                          2013046575

British Library Cataloguing in Publication Data
A CIP catalogue record for this book is available from the British Library

ISBN 978 1 84819 125 9
eISBN 978 0 85701 171 8

Printed and bound in Great Britain

CONTENTS

Part III An Experiential Programme of Study

ACKNOWLEDGEMENTS

Listening to Scent: An Olfactory Journey with Aromatic Plants and Their Extracts has been inspired and informed by those who guided me, formally and informally over the years, on the path to appreciating aromatic plant extracts and creating my own internal olfactory landscape, and also by *mon-koh*, or 'listening to fragrance'.

I would like to acknowledge my teachers and mentors, especially the late David Williams, whose willingness to educate aromatherapists as well as perfumers paved the way for further studies; and Tony Curtis, my tutor on the IFEAT (International Federation of Essential Oils and Aroma Trades) Diploma, who guided me through olfactory exercises and introduced me to a hitherto unknown realm of aromatics, both naturally derived and synthetic. Although I did not complete the Diploma, which I commenced in the early 1990s, I learned more about olfactory perception and communication than I could ever have imagined. Such is the power of building an olfactory memory! I regret now that I was unable to complete, but I have absolutely no regrets about undertaking the course. David Williams has left us a wonderful literary legacy, and Tony Curtis remains involved in perfumery education, now based at the University of Plymouth.

My 'formal' perfumery education stalled for many years; however, I remained personally and professionally active in the essential oil arena, and so I would also like to acknowledge the many writers whose words on aroma speak volumes to me – especially Robert Tisserand, Julia Lawless, Peter Holmes and Christopher McMahon, and the bloggers Denyse Beaulieu and Octavian Coifan. There are many more excellent authors, but, on reflection, these particular ones have probably had the greatest impact on me over the years. In 2012, I took the opportunity to continue with perfumery studies – I had wanted to do this for some time, not because I was under any illusions about entering the profession, but simply because I wanted to reconnect with fragrance composition. This time, it was a short course in artisan perfumery with the late Alec Lawless, and it would be fair to say that this special experience gave me a fresh and exciting perspective on scent creation, which has remained with me ever since. So thank you, Alec, you are missed by many, and I fully acknowledge your influence and legacy. I would also like to express my gratitude to my olfactory companions, in particular Audrey Quinn.

My husband Derek is responsible for the cover image – a favourite, intensely and heavily fragrant lily that has followed me around the country since my childhood – and also the colour images in the centre of the book, which capture just some of our olfactory adventures in France and the west coast of Scotland. Thank you, Derek, for your love and companionship, and for contributing to the book in a way that helps us to contextualise scents.

Finally, and as always, I would like to thank Singing Dragon – Jessica Kingsley, Jane Evans, Victoria Peters, Alex Fleming and Iona Twiston-Davies – for their professionalism, unfailing support and their willingness to take on novel projects such as this, and the copyeditor, Anne Oppenheimer.

Part I

LISTENING TO SCENT

1

Why Cultivate Your Sense of Smell?

Although many of us actively use our sense of smell, and very often enjoy the sensations it brings, relatively few of us take the time to educate and develop our olfactory palate. The rise in popularity of aromatherapy has indisputably brought an awareness of the benefits of the scents of essential oils, and the internet has certainly enabled perfume lovers to learn about fragrances and discuss them freely and without inhibitions. Structured training of the 'nose' is usually reserved for those entering a career in the fragrance industry. This process has inherent benefits, such as promoting olfactory awareness, developing discriminatory ability and acquiring an olfactory memory. Clearly these attributes are absolutely essential if the individual works with aromatic plant extracts. However, as we shall discover, the very process itself is therapeutic and enjoyable, and anyone who is interested in the sense of smell, fragrance, aromatherapy or natural perfumery can educate their nose too, and reap the benefits.

Here, we will learn to develop our olfactory vocabulary, experience the fragrances of aromatic plants and their extracts, and undertake exercises designed to facilitate odour recognition and discrimination. This will enable us to begin to acquire an olfactory memory. It is believed that cultivating the olfactory palate in this way can enhance our cognitive processes,[1] and can promote wellbeing. Additionally, it may mean that as we age and lose olfactory acuity (which invariably has a negative impact on wellbeing) our olfactory memory will help offset this loss. If we continue to consciously and actively use our sense of smell as we grow older, we might also keep its neural circuits

---

1 Cognition comes from the Latin word *cognosco* (*con* means 'with', and *gnosco* means 'know'). The word relates to the mental processes involved in the gaining of knowledge and understanding, through thought, experience and the senses. So the concept of cognition embraces perception, awareness, discernment, learning, insight, reasoning and thinking – all qualities and attributes essential when developing the olfactory palate.

active, and lessen the impact of time. The loss of the sense of smell is devastating at any stage of our lives, and no less so as time diminishes it.

As well as following a path that in some ways resembles that of a novice perfumer, we will discover that the journey need not be a solo one, unless, of course, that is what is preferred or necessary. Inspired by the Japanese art of *koh-do*, the 'way of incense', and its variation known as *kumikoh*, some group exercises have been devised. These will be equally suitable for professionals, such as aromatherapists and natural perfumers, and students or enthusiasts. Experiential learning of this type, where you are working with your senses, cognitive abilities and creative abilities, with like-minded individuals, can progress the deepest form of understanding. However, when your mind and senses are harnessed together in such enjoyable and creative tasks, you find that you can be 'in the moment', and so it is also possible to experience a real sense of wellbeing.

So there is a little bit of preparatory work to do before taking the first steps, but every single step that you take along the path represents real progress. It is my sincere hope you will find it interesting, challenging, fun and life-enhancing.

2

The Language of Scent

The first steps on the journey require familiarity with the vocabulary used in odour description, and then matching this with direct experience of the many odour types and their individual characteristics. Odour vocabulary is borrowed and adapted from that of the other senses, and indeed the arts, because in the English language there are no words exclusively reserved for the verbal or written communication of scents.

The language of scent is thus rich and evocative – and hearing or reading the words and phrases can conjure up a myriad of imaginary olfactory impressions. We will encounter words that identify the possible and actual sources of fragrances, and adjectives that further convey the nature of their impressions. It is also going to be helpful to recognise some of the words used by perfumers, which originated in the world of music. Beginning with the perfumer Septimus Piesse, who gave us the idea of 'notes', where aromatic extracts were matched along a musical scale, other musical terms entered the perfumer's vocabulary. These included 'chords' or 'accords', meaning combinations of odours that give a specific olfactory effect, just as a combination of musical notes gives a specific sound when they are delivered simultaneously. The perfumer's 'organ' is another example; this is a traditional piece of furniture reminiscent of a musical organ, constructed to house the many aromatic raw materials, arranged according to their notes, types and characteristics (see Colour Plate 1: The perfumer's organ at the Château de Chamerolles in France). Even the creation of a fragrance is known as 'composing' – in much the same way as a musician would compose a piece of music.

The olfactory language also reveals the extensive 'cross-modal' associations of scents: our sense of smell acquires inextricable associations with our other senses of taste, sight, hearing and touch. However, it is the close connection with taste that most often colours our perceptions and influences the way in which we describe odours.

For example, the scent of vanilla is invariably perceived and described as 'sweet', because of its associations with confections such as ice cream. In reality, vanilla does not taste sweet – if you pinch your nostrils together and chew a vanilla pod, your taste receptors will not detect a sweet element! Moreover, we usually encounter smells in a specific context. Thus, apart from tastes and flavours, scents can be associated with textures, sounds, music, shapes, colours and specific or diffuse feelings, and personal memories, and in this way our attempts at describing them can be communicated and our experiences shared.

Odour descriptions are complex, and the way in which odour vocabulary is used by untrained individuals can be very variable. Therefore it is important to learn to use the generally accepted vocabulary when defining olfactory impressions – we need to be consistent and accurate. We can learn to recognise odour 'types' and then qualify these with adjectives that begin to flesh out their individual characteristics. We can also learn to identify whether they are 'top notes' that evaporate quickly, or 'base notes' that are much slower to evaporate and persist, or whether they fall in between the two, the 'middle notes'. However, by considering their other properties such as intensity, their diffusiveness or how they fill the space, and how their scents change over time, we can then begin to build an accurate and meaningful odour profile – one that is not only defining, but also conveys the uniqueness of each and every one. It is also important to be neutral and objective. There will always be scents that attract us and some that do not, and some that we might dislike. This is perfectly normal, but strong emotional responses do not have relevance when constructing an odour description.

Please see Appendix 1, 'Odour Types and Characteristics Encountered in Aromatic Plant Extracts', for an explanation of the scent types and characteristics that you will encounter. This has all of the commonly used descriptive terms, and can be used as a starting point and quick reminder as you progress.

In the practice of perfumery, aromatic materials are also classified, so that their similarities, differences and interrelationships can be explored. Over centuries, probably beginning with the philosopher Aristotle (384–322 BCE), many schemes of classification have been proposed. The scheme proposed in 1960 by Steffen Arctander is generally recognised to be the most comprehensive classification of natural aromatics, as it attempts to define the relationships between

88 groups of over 400 materials. However, as Zarzo and Stanton (2009) commented, there is not, as yet, a universally agreed sensory map of odour descriptors. There is a good consensus of opinion; but because we cannot measure or assess odours objectively with instruments, but only subjectively with our noses, there will always be discrepancies and debate.

3

Our Olfactory System and its Connections

Before we go on to look at what educating our sense of smell might involve, and how it can bring benefits to our life, it makes sense to gain a basic understanding of how we detect and perceive odours, and how they can impact on our brain. We do have a reasonable understanding of the anatomy of our olfactory system (see Colour Plate 2) but much of its physiology remains theoretical. The following paragraph outlines what happens when we are exposed to an odour.

First, an odour exists in the form of a vapour – where its molecules are light enough to evaporate into the atmosphere and reach the nose. The *olfactory organ* is our detection system. This consists of very thin, twin membranes located on each side of the bony part of the nasal septum. It is thought that it contains around 800 million nerve endings, known as *olfactory hairs*. These are connected with the secondary neurons of the adjacent structure called the *olfactory bulb*, which extends to form the *olfactory nerve* (Williams 2000). Via the olfactory nerve tract, an olfactory signal is transmitted to the brain. Neurons from the olfactory tract project to several parts of the brain that constitute the *limbic system* (*limbus* means 'border'). The limbic system is situated in the temporal lobes of the brain; it is a diffuse region that is associated with emotional response, memories, motivation and pleasure – and where there is no conscious control. It comprises a loop of structures surrounding parts of the brain known as the *corpus callosum*. The neurons from the olfactory tract therefore project to the thalamus, where sensory integration occurs, the *hypothalamus*, where bodily functions are monitored and maintained, the *amygdala*, which is associated with basic emotions, and the *hippocampus*, which is associated with memory. In addition, the olfactory neurons also project into the *frontal cortex*, a region associated with organising and planning, where recognition of the odour occurs. The area known as the *prefrontal cortex* (PFC) is also influenced by odours – and this is where executive, logical and social decisions are made.

There are many connections between these parts of the brain. So there are two interrelated responses to odour – the cognitive, interpretative aspects at the frontal cortex and the emotional response at the limbic system. A smell can trigger emotional and physical reactions even without our conscious awareness of it. Olfactory signals, unlike other sensory inputs, do not always have to pass through the thalamus to reach the cerebral cortex. However, there is another aspect to the sense of smell that differs from the other senses in terms of brain connections. Olfaction is the only sense that does not to have a 'crossover' brain connection, so odours that enter the left nostril are accessed by the left hemisphere, while those entering the right will be accessed by the right hemisphere (Carter 2010; Hawkes and Doty 2009; Malaspina, Corcoran and Goudsmit 2006). This too has implications for how odours interact with the brain; for example, it was found that if the left nostril was occluded, the sympathetic nervous system predominated, and occlusion of the right nostril allowed predominance of the parasympathetic nervous system.[1] Also, in very loose terms, it is believed that the left hemisphere is associated with logic and analysis, and that the right hemisphere has a more sensory and artistic orientation. It is possible to assess how odours affect different areas of our brains by using Functional Magnetic Resonance Imaging (*f*MRI) scans, and these have revealed that brain activity can be considerable, even when the odours presented are at levels below our conscious detection (Hawkes and Doty 2009).

So although there is much that we do not yet understand about olfaction – such as how odour molecules bind to the olfactory receptor cells, or indeed how olfactory signals are generated, or how odour is interpreted by the brain, or the many factors that affect sensitivity – we do know that there is a direct and significant link between odours and our brains. Quinn (2012) discusses how brain development might be affected by olfaction (see also Bitter *et al.* 2010), and how some substances, such as inhaled recreational drugs and environmental toxins and pollutants, may even be related to the formation of dementia-related diseases, or possible catalysts for Alzheimer's and

---

1   The sympathetic and parasympathetic nervous systems are two of the three branches of the autonomic nervous system; the sympathetic system controls the internal organs, and the parasympathetic system controls the rest and relaxation responses.

Parkinson's disease, citing Doty (2009), Genter, Kendig and Knutson (2009), Hawkes *et al.* (2009) and Prediger *et al.* (2009). She also draws our attention to how hyposmia – a diminished sense of smell – may be an early indicator for Alzheimer's and Parkinson's disease, citing the studies of Bahar-Fuchs *et al.* (2011), Damholdt *et al.* (2011) and Morely *et al.* (2011).

4

Olfactory Sensitivity and Perception

At the outset it is important to realise that from birth we have a fully functional olfactory system. However, there are physiological and genetic factors which can be responsible for variations in the ability to detect and perceive odours. In addition to the ageing process diminishing olfactory sensitivity, some psychiatric disorders which feature depressive components can also affect olfactory perception (Lombion-Pouthier *et al.* 2006).

To educate the olfactory palate, you do not need to have an exceptional degree of sensitivity; a 'normal' nose is perfectly adequate. Perfumers have a greater degree of acuity than most novices, since they have worked with the sense of smell. However, research has shown that novices can quickly increase their olfactory sensitivity, simply by being repeatedly exposed to single odorants (Dalton and Wysocki 1996; Rabin and Cain 1986, cited in Dalton 1996; Semb 1968). So with regular, conscious exposure to scents, the perceived gap in sensitivity between perfumers and novices can be reduced very quickly.

Many individuals, including perfumers, have olfactory 'blind spots'. For example, Stansfield (2012) notes that around 50 per cent of adults cannot detect the odour of the hormone androsterone, found in human perspiration, even when it is presented at artificially high levels. Amongst those that can detect it, 15 per cent describe it as smelling like rubbing alcohol. Another phenomenon is 'partial anosmia'.[1] This is the term used to describe the situation where an individual has difficulty in perceiving or cannot detect certain odorants. Calkin and Jellinek (1994) suggest that even some very skilful perfumers are not able to smell specific perfumery materials such as musks, woody odorants or aromachemicals in their pure form, but they can detect their effects within a composition.

---

1   Anosmia is loss of the sense of smell.

5

Discrimination

Sensitivity to odours can be understood in two ways. The first, as noted above, is the ability to detect odours, even at very low concentrations. This is known as the 'detection threshold'. The second is the 'recognition threshold' – the lowest concentration at which an odour can be described, or discriminated from another odour (Laska and Ringh 2010). Compared with the ability to detect, there is more variation in the ability to discriminate. One of the biggest differences between novices and perfumers is the ability of the latter to discriminate between odours when they are presented in a mixture (Livermore and Laing 1996).

Barkat *et al.* (2012) commented that in natural conditions our olfactory systems are normally required to process complex odours all of the time, because most of the odours we are exposed to are in fact composed of several or even many odorants. This means that our olfactory receptors must interact with neural processing of the signals generated by these mixtures. However, Barkat *et al.* suggest that the perception of a mixture is not simply the sum of its components; and indeed, if more than four components are involved, new odour sensations can be produced. This phenomenon can be seen in perfumery. For example, Burr (2007) relates an interview with the perfumer Jean-Claude Ellena, who is renowned for his ability to work with comparatively few ingredients. During this interview Ellena demonstrated that if the sweet, chamomile-like chemical known as *iso*-butyl phenylacetate is combined with synthetic vanilla (ethyl vanillin), the mixture smells like chocolate, which itself contains around 800 odorous molecules. The same ethyl vanillin with cinnamon, orange and lime essences can replicate the smell of 'coca cola'. Barkat *et al.* (2012) suggest that this might be because mixtures can stimulate olfactory neurons which are not stimulated by the individual odorants within the mixture.

Returning to the concept of olfactory discrimination, we must also consider another important factor, and that is the ability to give a verbal label to odour perceptions. This too can be learned. In 1996 Dalton and Wysocki studied longer-term adaptation to odours, and demonstrated that repeated exposure to single odours, *in conjunction with standard odour descriptors and qualities*, can enhance the ability to verbalise olfactory perceptions. The only way to develop this ability is to practise. So although some work is involved, the effects go beyond simply learning how to discriminate and describe scents. By doing this, we are in fact joining cognition with sensory processing, and developing an odour memory.

6

Olfactory Memory and the Reasoning Processes

Without doubt, the single biggest difference between novices and perfumers is in olfactory memory and, directly related to this, the considerable cognitive skills involved in composing fragrances. The highly influential perfumer Jean Carles (1892–1966), who composed the classic fragrance *Tabu* in 1931, highlighted the importance of olfactory memory. When his sense of smell declined he could still work by drawing on his olfactory memory, composing the successful *Ma Griffe* in 1945 and collaborating on *Miss Dior* in 1947.

It has been suggested that it takes at least ten years of creative activity to develop expertise as a perfumer, over and above the time devoted to educating the nose. However, here the goal is not to train and practise as a perfumer, but to work actively with the olfactory palate, because of the inherent benefits in doing so. We will not only be stimulating our senses, but also developing our reasoning[1] processes.

The reasoning process is one of the highest cognitive functions and takes place in the prefrontal cortex[2] (PFC) of the brain. This is the area associated with making 'executive' decisions, planning, and orchestrating our thoughts, actions and social interactions; and it is sometimes said to be associated with positive emotion. Fujii *et al.* (2007), using near infrared spectroscopy,[3] examined the prefrontal activity of *koh-do* masters (experts) and novices during an incense discrimination task. They found with the masters that the first inhalation, when the first impression of the scent is formed, provides

---

1   Reasoning is the process of using our knowledge to reach conclusions, or construct explanations for what we observe.

2   The prefrontal cortex is located in the anterior (i.e. the front) portion of the frontal cortex.

3   This is a technique using the near infrared part of the electromagnetic spectrum that allows non-invasive assessment of brain function. It can monitor blood flow, blood oxygenation and neural activity.

names and mental 'images' to both the left and right areas of the PFC. Then, during the discrimination phase, the PFC shapes and sorts these images, and sends a query to the knowledge base, to find the name or an associated image. When the response is received, the answer is then compared with the image still being generated by the incense stimulus. This final processing takes place by communication between the left PFC, which retrieves the name, and the right PFC, which is concerned with the shape of the image, until the best conclusion is reached. This is an example of abductive reasoning,[4] where a conclusion is drawn from multiple premises. Novices appeared to have more difficulty in reasoning about the olfactory stimulus, because they did not show these dynamic and organised PFC patterns. This might be because they did not have a prelearned knowledge base; or perhaps because, although they could create internal images, they could not represent these images in the symbolic space. In other words, they had not learned to manipulate abstract concepts. This research showed that the masters of *koh-do* had achieved the highest possible levels of cognitive processing. When the expert in perfumery is compared with the *koh-do* master, we can see many parallels, especially in terms of discrimination, olfactory memory and creativity. It is suggested, therefore, that an expert perfumer is also capable of the highest level of cognitive processing – abductive reasoning – and that taking steps to cultivate our olfactory palate will also improve our cognitive functioning.

Lawless (2010) compared the experience of smelling with 'awareness and enquiry' with the 'just sitting' method of meditation. He explained that this method is a practice of body awareness known as *shikantaza*, which is attributed to the Zen master Dogen. In order

---

4   There are three types of reasoning. *Deductive* reasoning is based on a general premise of rule, and is a logical sequence of thoughts that leads to a 'sound or false' conclusion. This allows observations to be made and implications to be defined, but deductive reasoning is not predictive. *Inductive* reasoning is based on specific and limited observations, and leads to a general conclusion. Very often scientific research is inductive, as it involves gathering data or evidence and looking for patterns or trends, so that a hypothesis which explains the observations can be formed. The conclusion is not certain, but can contribute to our knowledge base, and it can be predictive. In contrast, *abductive* reasoning is based on incomplete observations, and progresses towards the most likely explanation for these observations. A medical diagnosis or the conclusion reached by a jury in a court case are examples of the abductive reasoning process, as were Einstein's 'thought experiments'; abductive reasoning is thus creative and intuitive (Butte College, no date).

to still the mind, awareness is deliberately shifted to the body, which is always 'present', unlike our thoughts, and, with practice, mind and body become harmonised. When we fully engage with a scent and it becomes our focus, we can detach from busy, distracting thoughts, what Bloom (2011) calls our 'monkey mind', and experience a state of mindfulness and reflective awareness.

So it is suggested here that working with our olfactory palate has threefold benefits – sensory, cognitive and emotional. It can stimulate our olfactory receptors and perhaps maintain acuity, it can improve our cognitive abilities and, not least, it can contribute to wellbeing.

7

The First Steps

The perfumer and theorist Edmond Roudnitska (1905–1996) was known for his respect for the scents of the natural world, and the way he used these as reference points for his compositions. For example, he would compare the scent of lily-of-the-valley flowers growing in his garden with blotters of his composition *Diorissimo* as it evolved. The perfumer Sandrine Videault, who was mentored by Roudnitska, referred to the flowers of *Gardenia tahitensis* (the beautiful Polynesian 'tiaré') when composing *Manoumalia*, and Calice Becker did likewise with tuberose when composing *Beyond Love* (Turin and Sanchez 2009). So even if you are already working with aromatic materials, it is always a good idea to begin with an exploration (or revisitation) of the aromas of natural plant materials, such as fresh and dried herbs, fruits, spices, wood, conifer needles, twigs and resins, and scented flowers. These are all easily accessed, and will provide most of the odour types and characteristics that are necessary for experiential learning. This is also the time to start keeping written records of all your sensory impressions.

Once the associations between the odour and its source have been made – that is, once the connections between sensory perception and a verbal label have been established – an olfactory memory has been created. When you feel ready, you can begin to attempt identification. This involves 'blind' sampling, where the aromatics are presented in the absence of visual identification and knowledge of the source; and this will obviously require assistance from a friend or colleague. Again, keep a note of your progress.

A systematic approach to sampling aromatic plant materials, coupled with keeping records of your sensory impressions, gives a very good base from which to explore the aromas of essential oils and absolutes. These are much more 'concentrated' and intense aromas, and often do not smell like their natural counterparts until diluted. Essential oils are usually liquids, although they vary in viscosity (thickness), from being less viscous than water, such as the citrus oils, to more viscous than water, such as sandalwood. Some absolutes have a thick liquid form, such as rose, jasmine and orange blossom. Others have a paste-like consistency, and some resinoids are hard and brittle, such as benzoin. These can be purchased as alcohol extraits[1] (a 10–30% concentration is ideal), or diluted in an odourless solvent such as dipropylene glycol (DPG); these preparations are also suitable for sensory exercises. Some of the paste-like absolutes can be gently warmed in a hot water-bath and this can make them more fluid, but ensure that they are tightly capped and dried before opening.

The supplier should be able to provide not only botanical authentication but also safety data for all products, and this should be checked and consulted before using aromatic extracts. Although we are concerned with the scents of the aromatic extracts, unintentional skin contact may occur, so, again, ensure that you have access to safety information. This is usually provided by the suppliers of essential oils (see the list at the end of the book) and may also be found in aromatherapy texts, such as Lawless (2012); however, for the aromatherapy practitioner or student it is worth investing in a dedicated text such as Tisserand and Young (2014).

---

1   *Extrait* is the French word for 'extract'. Originally, 'extrait' perfumes were produced by alcoholic extraction of enfleurage pomade (see glossary entry 'enfleurage'). The term came to describe strong alcoholic solutions of perfume compound (or indeed absolute or resinoid), and it is currently used to describe the strongest form of alcoholic perfume/extract that is commercially available (between 5 and 20% of perfume compound/extract in strong ethanol).

8

How to Conduct Sensory Exercises

Sensory exercises should be conducted in peace and quiet, and in an ordered and methodical manner. Everything that is required should be at hand, including your samples, blotters ('smelling strips'), notebook and pencil. Ideally, the environment should be warm, free of draughts, well ventilated, and away from other smells. It is also important to feel relaxed and comfortable before commencing. All aromatic extracts should be carefully applied to blotters, not sampled directly from the bottle. This is so that the different phases of fragrance can be appreciated, and this cannot be achieved otherwise. The blotter should always be labelled before use, with a reference and the time; it can be folded across its length to form a 45° bend at both ends to form a 'handle' and an elevated tip for the sample, so that it can be put aside without the sample touching anything else. The blotter can then be dipped in the aromatic extract, up to 0.5cm, or one drop can be dispensed on the tip. If an alcoholic extrait is being sampled, always wait for the alcohol to evaporate, as alcohol will temporarily 'numb' your olfactory receptors.

The smelling technique is important. The nose adapts to odours very quickly, so it is important to work quickly at first. Initial impressions should be gathered before fatigue sets in. The eyes should be closed to eliminate visual distractions, and your awareness should be directed to the odour. Sniff the sample (it is not necessary to inhale[1]), concentrate on the impressions, and record your perceptions of the top notes immediately. Check this from time to time over the next five minutes, looking for changes. The blotter can then be put aside, and a short break taken before assessing the next sample. The blotters

---

1   Prolonged inhalation of scents can influence the autonomic nervous system and elicit mental and emotional changes; here we are concerned with their olfactory characteristics. Additionally, the rate of airflow in the nostrils can determine substance absorption levels (Hawkes and Doty 2009); this may also have a direct impact on which elements of aroma are detected (Quinn 2012).

should be returned to at intervals (15 minutes and 45 minutes) to assess the different notes, looking for the body and dryout phases.[2] In the case of the citrus oils, the body notes will emerge very quickly and the dryout will be barely perceptible, even after just 30 minutes. The body notes of other oils, typically those classed as middle notes, will begin to emerge after 15–45 minutes, and their dryouts after anywhere between 90 minutes and several hours. However, the dryouts of the base notes, such as sandalwood and vetiver, will be present on the smelling strip for several days. So the sampling time should be managed accordingly. In each session it is best to limit the sampling to two or three materials.

It is also possible to 'fatigue' your nose to top notes just before smelling the middle notes, or to fatigue your nose to the middle notes before smelling base notes, and by doing this you can achieve more clarity in each phase. This sounds complicated, but in fact it is quite straightforward. The following method was used in perfumery education. It is not suggested that you routinely apply this technique, but it is interesting to try it out once or twice.

1. Label a blotter with the name of your aromatic and the reference 'Dip 1'.

2. Fold the blotter as described above.

3. Dip the blotter in the essential oil or absolute, or place two or three drops on the tip (or an equivalent smear if the extract is paste-like).

4. Make a note of the time.

5. Smell carefully, noting your initial impressions. Relate these to the odour type (e.g. floral, woody, citrus) and characteristics (fresh, warm, rich, etc.).

6. Return to Dip 1 over the next five minutes, and see if you can detect any changes – make a note of these.

7. Label a second blotter with the name and reference Dip 2, and prepare a second dip as in step 3 above. Note the time, and focus on smelling Dip 2.

---

2   The body notes are the 'heart' of the scent, given by constituents of moderate volatility, but influenced by the top notes as they fade, and also the least volatile constituents that form the base notes, as they begin to evaporate. The dryout (or drydown) is the odour that remains after the top and middle notes have evaporated.

8. Immediately compare the fresh Dip 2 with Dip 1, which will now be about 15 minutes old. The two blotters will smell very different. What new characteristics have emerged in Dip 1? Have the original notes changed, faded, or become more intense? Dip 2 will give an olfactory impression of the top notes, while Dip 1 will show you the body notes. Make a note of your perceptions.

9. Set both strips aside for 45 minutes.

10. Return to Dip 1, and look for further changes. Use Dip 2 as a comparison.

11. The 'dryout' notes will begin to emerge after anywhere between 90 minutes and two hours. The odour of some aromatics, particularly the 'base' notes, can persist for several days, because of their comparatively low volatility.

This exercise will give you a very good idea of how the nose behaves; it will give you first-hand experience of how the scent of an essential oil or absolute develops over time, and a deeper understanding of what we mean by top, body and dryout notes.

By this stage, you will be well prepared to commence some structured sensory exercises that will lead to enhanced discrimination and the ability to verbalise your perceptions of odour.

9

Odour Families, Types
and Characteristics

There are several classification schemes whereby odours can be placed within broad categories, or 'families'. Most of the readily available aromatic plant extracts are placed in the following families, and the odour profiles are organised within these groupings:

- balsamic
- woody
- spicy
- coniferous
- herbaceous
- medicated
- green
- agrestic
- floral
- fruity
- citrus (sometimes called hesperidic).

As we shall quickly discover, some of them contain 'sub-families', and there are a few aromatics, such as patchouli and blackcurrant bud, that are so complex and distinctive that they almost defy categorisation. The artisan perfumer, Alec Lawless, suggested that these belong to the 'maverick' family (Lawless 2009)!

So when learning about odour types and characteristics, it is best that the process is carefully structured by selecting samples which have the attributes for a particular set or family of scents. For example, when exploring the woody family, you could choose Virginian cedar as your 'reference' for wood, and let this enter your olfactory memory, complete with its characteristics. Other woods, such as sandalwood and guaiacwood, can then be sampled, noting their differing characteristics. Olfactory impressions should be recorded using the standard odour vocabulary to identify the different characteristics. The process cannot be rushed. The aim is to determine the dynamic 'personality' of each scent – its character, duration, and how it evolves over time. However, you should also be aware of any personal associations with particular scents, because this is another way of tapping into your olfactory memory. The goals, apart from pleasure, are to learn to smell with awareness, to stimulate the olfactory receptors and to build an olfactory memory.

It does not really matter which family you begin with, but you might like to work from the balsams – often base notes – to the woods, the spicy family, then the coniferous, herbaceous, medicated, green, agrestic and floral families, the fruity family and the related citrus family, which is more representative of top notes. The odour profiles in Part II are organised into these families, with botanical sources, odour descriptors, olfactory notes and suggestions for comparisons. *It is not expected that you should obtain all of the aromatics in the first instance.* Some of the recommended suppliers may be able to supply custom-made collections if requested, but bear in mind that availability, quality and costs fluctuate.

A short introduction to the families follows below.

Balsamic family (profiles: labdanum, opopanax, tolu balsam and vanilla)

In this family you will find several 'sub-families'. The vanilla type is typified by vanilla absolute, but you might also want to sample some benzoin resinoid, which contains the vanilla-scented constituent vanillin (an aromatic aldehyde – see Glossary and Appendix 2). Tolu balsam, although it also contains a small amount of vanillin, is an example of the cinnamate type, where constituents known as cinnamyl alcohol and cinnamic acid are responsible for a warm, heavy and balsamic, cinnamon-like effect, with a fruity strawberry-like note. Some balsamic scents, such as labdanum, have an ambra nature.

'Ambra' is the term used to denote an ambergris-like odour[1] – a scent that is difficult to define, but is complex, rich, musty, musky, earthy and ambery. Finally, because of their distinctive spicy characteristics, opopanax and myrrh are always said to be at the 'far end' of the balsamic spectrum (Curtis and Williams 2009; Lawless 2009). The sweet, chocolate-like cacao absolute could also be classed as a balsamic scent – but without any vanilla nuances.

Woody family (profiles: guaiacwood, sandalwood and Virginian cedarwood)

The woody family is comprised of the exotic or 'precious' woods – those that are valued for their fragrances and use in carving, the rosy-scented woods and the woods of some conifers. The most valued of the woody scents must be that of true sandalwood (*Santalum album*), and this is now very scarce, but if you can obtain the essential oil, do take the chance to compare it with the more readily available *S. austrocaledonicum* and *S. spicatum*. Erligmann (2001) classifies *S. album* as amber-like and *S. spicatum* as resinous. As for *S. austrocaledonicum*, less is known about its constituents and their contribution to the odour profile, but it is certainly more amber-like than resinous. Virginian cedarwood is possibly the most 'typical' of the woody odour type – and here you will find a slight resinous quality. Guaiacwood represents the rosy aspect in the woody family, which you will also find in rosewood.

Spicy family (profiles: caraway seed, carrot seed, clove bud and nutmeg)

This family is, as you would expect, populated by the scents of culinary spices – warm, pungent, sometimes earthy, sometimes woody, sometimes fresh, fruity or even sweet. Clove bud and cinnamon leaf are typical – both have a fruity character. Caraway seed is also typically

---

1   Ambergris is a substance secreted by some whales when indigestible cuttlefish 'beaks' lodge in their intestines. If it passes through the gut and is released into the sea, this unpleasant-smelling secretion rises to the surface, and the action of sun, waves and salt water transforms it into a beautiful-smelling substance. This can be found washed up on beaches, and was an important perfumery material. It is rare, and more costly than gold.

warm and spicy, but very distinctive, as is carrot seed with its sweet, woody and fresh/earthy nature. Nutmeg is an example of a woody spicy scent which also has a sweet, ethereal nature.

The spicy family is large, and there are other members that you might like to sample. Fenugreek is unusual because, although it is certainly spicy, reminiscent of curry, very rich and warm, it also displays celery-like and walnut-like facets. Celery seed is another warm and spicy member of this family, while cumin seed has an interesting but not entirely unpleasant note reminiscent of an 'unwashed body odour'. The Asian mint, *Perilla frutescens* (shiso mint) also has a very complex odour in which you might pick up on caraway and cumin notes.

Coniferous family (profiles: Scots pine and Siberian fir)

The coniferous family is easily identified by the familiar aromatic, woody scent of pine, and also the resinous nature of pine (*Pinus* species), spruce (*Picea* species) and fir (*Abies* species) essential oils. The coniferous/resinous odour is reminiscent of the forest, and the essential oils may have balsamic notes too. The main constituents of the coniferous oils are α- and β-pinenes, which are chemicals classed as monoterpenes, and so you might also be able to detect a pine-like, 'terpeney' note.

Herbaceous family (profiles: clary sage, laurel leaf, lavender and thyme)

In perfumery terms, sage would constitute a typical herbaceous odour – although some individuals perceive this as urinous! However, just as with the spicy family, you will find many nuances and sub-families. Lavender (the essential oils of *Lavandula* species, but not lavender absolute, which is floral) is one sub-family; camphoraceous (rosemary essential oil), tea (clary sage essential oil), minty (*Mentha* species) and thymolic (common thyme essential oil) are others. Camphoraceous, minty, mentholic and thymolic odours are also classed as medicated. However, by smelling the herbal *absolutes* for comparison, we can begin to understand the value of the herbaceous family in perfumery, because these herbal odours are closer to the natural sources than their essential oils, which so often have medicated natures.

Medicated family (profiles: eucalyptus, peppermint and wintergreen)

Medicated odours are associated with traditional medicines – especially liniments for exterior use – and have a penetrating nature. They are rarely used in perfumery. White camphor can represent the camphoraceous note, while eucalyptus blue gum typifies the cineolic[2] odour type, also found in many other eucalypts and some paperbarks. Peppermint represents the 'cooling' mentholic sub-family, and juniperberry is terpenic (its main constituents are monoterpenes, which give this particular effect). Wintergreen is so distinctive that it has its own category, defined by its main constituent methyl salicylate, which can also be detected in the intensely floral ylang ylang extra.

Green family (profiles: violet leaf and galbanum)

The green odour type, which is reminiscent of crushed green foliage, is often noted as a sub-family within complex odours, and can be represented by violet leaf absolute and galbanum essential oil. Violet leaf has an intense, green scent, while galbanum is also intense, but is less leafy and more like freshly podded peas, or chopped green peppers.

Agrestic family (profiles: hay, oakmoss, patchouli and tobacco leaf)

The term 'agrestic' refers to odours that are in some way reminiscent of the countryside or the great outdoors – woods, meadows, damp earth. Here we find the complex mossy scent of oakmoss and tree moss absolutes, the grassy smell of flouve essential oil or foin absolute, the new-mown hay effect of tonka bean absolute (imparted by a constituent called coumarin) and the sweet, rich hay absolute. Vetiver essential oil could represent the earthy aspect of the agrestic family, as could patchouli, and you might like to sample seaweed absolute to discover an odour of the seashore. Tobacco leaf absolute is rich and warm, and also represents the 'tabac' odour type.

---

2 'Cineolic' describes a penetrating eucalyptus-like odour, which gets its name from one of the principal chemical components of eucalyptus oil – 1,8-cineole.

Floral family (profiles: champaca, frangipani, genet, jasmine, linden blossom, mimosa, narcissus, orange blossom, osmanthus, pink lotus, rose and ylang ylang)

This is another big family, and one which is very important in perfumery. A floral scent is that of the living or freshly picked flower, and what we encounter in essential oils and absolutes can only be an approximation or illustration of 'floral' (Curtis and Williams 2009). As you can imagine, there is a wide variation within the floral category, from the rosy but herbaceous/green/minty geranium, to the green and delicate linden blossom and the heady, exotic, powerful ylang ylang. The floral scents can be elusive when attempts are made to categorise them; however, bearing this in mind, we could consider that there are several sub-groups. These are rose (rose itself, and rosy-scented extracts such as geranium, palmarosa and immortelle); indolic (meaning the heady scents of white flowers such as white lilac and lily,[3] jasmine, white champaca, tuberose and orange blossom); violet (represented by violet flower and orris root, but not included here because of cost and availability); narcotic (such as hyacinth and narcissus, and also lily); honey/hay-like (such as genet and broom); green and delicate (mimosa and linden); citrus-like (aglaia); fruity (osmanthus, frangipani and ylang ylang); earthy/green (narcissus) and earthy/leathery (pink lotus).

Fruity family (profiles: blackcurrant bud, Roman chamomile and tagetes)

The fruity note (that is, other than the citrus sub-family) is represented in a few aromatic plant extracts; here include the fruity/green and 'catty' blackcurrant bud, and the apple-like, herbaceous tagetes. A fruity apple note is also found in Roman chamomile essential oil.

Citrus family (profiles: bergamot, cédrat, mandarin and Litsea cubeba)

The large citrus family can be represented by the typical citrus scent of cédrat, the floral, peppery citrus scent of bergamot and the complex

---

3 Many flowers, including white lilac and lily, do not yield essential oils or absolutes, despite their distinctive scents.

and soft nature of mandarin. However, some non-citrus fruit-derived aromatics such as *Litsea cubeba* have a pronounced lemony note, so these have also been included in the citrus odour family. This family is sometimes called the hesperidic family.

A suggested programme of study, based on aromatics in the natural world and the olfactory profiles in Part II, is presented in Part III. Work your way through your selection of aromatics, and feel free to return to each one as you wish. This will help consolidate your perceptions and your ability to recognise the odour types and characteristics. You can also begin to compare and contrast scents from different families. The process cannot be rushed! You can travel solo for this part of the journey, but sometimes having a companion to share the experiences can be helpful. Also, if you join forces with other like-minded individuals, the cost of the aromatics can be shared, and a wider range can be accessed.

However, to take the next steps, explained in Chapter 10, you will need assistance, and if you can find 'scent companions', so much the better…

10

The Next Steps

Identification and Discrimination

Just as with the natural plant materials, your progress with identification can be assessed with assisted blind sampling. If you close your eyes and a blotter is presented to you, can you describe the attributes of the odour, and perhaps name it? Again, record keeping is important, of errors as well as successful identifications.

The 'odd man out' test (or 'triangle test') can test the ability to discriminate between odours. The simplest way of carrying this out is to have someone prepare three blotters, each labelled with a code and the numbers 1, 2 and 3. Two of the blotters should have the same sample applied, and the third should be different – but not too different, and from the same olfactory family. When you are presented with the blotters, can you tell which two are the same and which one is different? Can you describe the difference? Can you identify the samples?

Once you are further along the olfactory path, you might want to explore what happens with different combinations of oils and absolutes. For some ideas, see Appendix 3, 'Building Accords'. You can start with simple binary combinations ('duos') – prepared by putting three drops of each of two oils in a small, clean bottle. Dip the blotter, let it absorb, and see what you perceive. It will probably be fairly easy to sense some of the characteristics of the two components. With help, this can be done 'blind': ask someone to prepare a combination that is unknown to you – can you discriminate, can you identify the components? Then you can begin to explore what happens with mixtures of three or more oils. In Roudnitska's words:

> When introduced into a mixture, the odour ceases to be one entity and interacts freely with other odorous bodies. Take note of everything that comes to mind, using the words which arise naturally; if they enable a thought to be more precise, if they surround the contours of the odours without ambiguity. Avoid

'almost' at any cost. Try to find the words that unequivocally define the impression so that twenty years later, if confronted with the same impression, the same words come to mind. (Roudnitska 1991, cited by Aftel 2008, pp.60–61)

Bear in mind that the scent of each essential oil or absolute, and indeed each aromatic plant, is given by many constituents, each of which has its own characteristics, and their relative proportions will also have a major impact on the aroma. So the whole scent is something much, much more than the sum of its constituents. When the already complex essential oils and absolutes are combined, the potential for creating new effects is vast. However, it is not only the combinations of ingredients but also their ratios (relative proportions) that will determine the nature of the new aroma. In reality the potential for creating new fragrances is infinite. Moreover, the process of creation, which involves active olfaction, and complete focus on scent, can have effects which can be compared to concentrative meditation. It can, in fact, be very therapeutic!

11

Creative Blending

When discussing creative blending, Lawless (2009) emphasised that we must be thoroughly familiar with our essential oils and absolutes, saying that 'deep familiarity with them is the ground which can feed the roots of inspiration' (p.55). He also made the pertinent observation that we need to work with our instinctual nature too. Although fragrance composition is beyond the scope of this particular sensory journey, an insight into how 'natural' perfumes are structured can underpin creativity. Calkin and Jellinek (1994) highlight several important principles; most importantly, that a perfume is not composed randomly, but is the result of a precise system of structures, based on:

> the precise olfactory relationship between individual ingredients, known as the 'perfumery accord', the relationship between simplicity and complexity, and the balance between materials of different volatility suitable for the product for which the perfume is intended. (p.13)

Jean Carles constructed base accords with materials of low volatility, middle or modifying accords with ingredients of medium volatility, and top note accords which included the more volatile ingredients. He would then experiment extensively, to explore, define and record the olfactory effects given by combining various ratios of the three accords.

It is a good exercise to compose some accords on paper, because this will allow you to think about the possible relationships between the aromatics and how they might affect one another – their olfactory interplay. An accord can be made up of two or more aromatic materials and its effect will depend not only on the ingredients but also on their relative proportions (ratios). You can also think about combining accords with the intent of composing a simple fragrance.

To do this, first you will need to identify the theme of your composition. This might be something abstract, such as a season or a place or atmosphere, or perhaps simply a fragrance type or a specific essential oil or absolute. This will give you the first idea of the aromatic palette that you will be working with, and the heart of your idea. Then you need to consider the base, middle and top accords, and how these will relate to each other and might manifest in your final composition. Because the middle accord generally carries the main theme of the fragrance, this should be addressed first. However, the base accord will be the most persistent, and it will obviously affect the perception and evolution of the heart, and so should have some connection, or a 'bridge', to the middle accord. The top notes of a scent are always noticed first; they have an initial impact, and help lift the middle notes, but fade away eventually. However, they too should have a relationship with the heart of the fragrance, so we must consider the top–middle olfactory bridges too. We also need to remain cognisant of the odour intensity and diffusiveness of our materials. For a fuller exploration of how a natural fragrance can be created, see Chapter 6 of Lawless (2009).

See also Appendix 3, 'Building Accords', for some examples that you might like to experiment with.

12

In the Spirit of *Koh-do*

This olfactory journey, like many journeys, can be enhanced by travelling companions. The following activities are social; they are celebrations of scent which offer us a chance to play, appreciate and create.

Koh-do, the 'way of incense', is a Japanese art which originated in the Muromachi period (1336–1573 CE). Rather than using the popular *nerikoh* (blended balls, where incense is bound with honey or the flesh of plums), some individuals returned to the practice of burning jinkoh[1] (incense wood) on its own, and enjoying the scent. This eventually became known as 'listening' to incense, or *mon-koh*. The concept of listening to rather than smelling incense is interesting; in Buddha's realm everything is fragrant, including his words. Incense and fragrance are synonymous, and his words are therefore incense, which should be listened to. *Koh-do* was established by Ashikaga Yoshimasa, a patron of the arts, his adviser Shino Soshin, and Sanjonishi Sanetaka, a scholar who was in charge of incense at the imperial court. They classified the *jinkoh* and all of the available incenses at the court, and established the protocols and etiquette for incense appreciation, often linking it with literary themes. At the end of the Muromachi period, *koh-do* was an established art form, its popularity endured, and it was taught first by connoisseurs, who then established schools headed by professional masters of *koh-do*. In accordance with traditional Japanese practice, the teachings, including the spiritual and philosophical aspects, were kept secret, passed on by word of mouth, and only shared with proficient students. However, its popularity meant that *koh-do* also became like a game, the spiritual element was lost, and its popularity declined as 'westernisation'

---

1   Agarwood, the resin-rich wood of *Aquilaria* species, was the preferred incense wood; it is rare and very expensive, and its aroma is the result of the accumulation of a resin which is formed in response to accidental fungal infection.

increased. The *koh-do* revival began in the 1960s, and continues today in its native Japan, the USA and Europe (Morita 1992).

There is much in *koh-do* that we can apply to the sensory appreciation of aromatic plant extracts. We can use its structure to 'listen' to their scents, and because it is a social activity, our progress can be measured and our experiences can be shared with like-minded individuals. *Koh-do* presents us with a wonderful opportunity for collaborative learning.

Morita (1992) explains the fundamentals of the incense ceremony. The room should be big enough to accommodate ten people, including a master of ceremonies, a record keeper and eight participants. The participants sit on straw mats on the floor, according to a traditional seating arrangement. In the Shino School tradition the record keeper sits to the right of the master of ceremonies, while the participants sit clockwise from the master of ceremonies. The place to the left of the master is reserved for an honoured guest or an elderly participant. Once the participants are in place, the master and record keeper enter, both carrying specific paraphernalia related to incense burning and record keeping. The master then greets the participants, and formally explains the proceedings, which are governed by ancient and strict protocols. However, both the master and record keeper take part, while ensuring that the incense burning is in order. The record keeper, as you might expect, is also responsible for keeping records of the participants and their answers. After each activity, the record keeper should pass around the participants' answers, and these can be explored in a relaxed manner.

It is not suggested that when adapting this for sensory appreciation of plant aromatics we need to follow the same strict etiquette and protocols, but it certainly makes sense to have someone in the 'master of ceremonies' role, and another individual who will take responsibility for record keeping and paperwork. In any case, it is strongly suggested that the proceedings are well thought out beforehand, ordered, methodical, and explained clearly to all who are participating. The master of ceremonies should ideally be an experienced individual, but a reasonable knowledge of plant aromatics and their handling should be sufficient to fulfil this role, and the programme of study explained in this book will more than suffice. The participants will require at least a familiarity with odour vocabulary, and a mix of beginners and those more advanced in their studies is perfectly fine. It is not absolutely necessary to have eight participants – two, four or six will also work well.

Morita (1992) also tells us that the 'true spirit of *koh-do*... is really a party to appreciate and play with fragrances' (p.107). In Japan, art forms are often described as *asobi*, a word that translates as 'play'. Morita discusses the use of this word in relation to *koh-do*, and comments that one of the reasons for play is 'compensating for unfulfilled longing'. She also quotes the Dutch historian Johan Huizinga (1955), saying that:

> Play casts a spell over us: it is 'enchanting' and 'captivating' and brings us 'to rhythm and harmony'. (Morita 1992, p.103)

We could then argue that because beautiful scents can have similar effects on the psyche, 'play' is a perfect way to harness these benefits.

Apart from 'listening' to single aromatics, there are several activities that can be adapted from *koh-do*. *Kumikoh* are games that involve two or more types of incense, and some suggestions follow. Feel free to interpret and modify the themes and suggestions to suit your group – whether it is a gathering of scent lovers or an aromatherapy or artisan perfumery workshop.

In each case the record keeper could collect the answer sheets, and the data can be recorded electronically on a spreadsheet. This can then be sent to the participants following the gathering, and acts as a useful record of experience and progress. Each participant should be given small, re-sealable plastic bags or paper envelopes in which to place their blotters after use, or the blotters can be collected and sealed and removed from the area so that their scents do not interfere with subsequent exercises.

Listening – scent description and identification

Prior to the meeting, the master of ceremonies should decide on the aromatics to be listened to. Depending on other exercises planned, this could be between three and five. A blotter of each should be prepared for each participant, simply labelled from one to five. These should be passed to the participants, one sample at a time. The record keeper should give each participant a score sheet with space to write their name, the sample reference number, odour description and identity. The participants should be allowed 'quiet' time to note their impressions, including the odour family, subsidiary odour types, and the characteristics of the top and middle notes, before the second blotter is presented. After all of the samples have been listened to, the participants should be given a few minutes to revisit the samples to see if there are any further impressions, and whether they can give the aromatics an identity.

At the end of this exercise the identities and descriptions can be revealed and there can be a free exchange of impressions, after which the record keeper collects the answers.

Sanshu-koh (the game of three)

This is, essentially, the 'odd man out' or 'triangle test' which can give an indication of olfactory acuity and discrimination. The master of ceremonies should choose the scents, and can make this as difficult or easy as desired. Some suggestions are: geranium from different geographical regions (such as Réunion and China); two species of the same genus (e.g. *Santalum album* and *S. austrocaledonicum*); or the rosy/woody scented essential oils of guaiacwood and rosewood. For each pair of participants three blotters should be prepared, each labelled with a code and the numbers 1, 2 and 3. Each participant should be given a score sheet with space to write their name and answers. Two of the blotters should have the same sample applied, and the third should be different. The sets of three blotters should be given to pairs of participants, who can take turns at presenting them to their partner. The question is 'Which blotter is different – 1, 2 or 3?' Without conferring or speaking, the answers should be recorded. On completion, the identities of the scents can be revealed and discussed, and the answer sheets collected.

Naming accords

This exercise has two functions. It allows the participants to exercise their ability to identify odour families, and then test their discriminatory ability. Prior to the gathering, the master of ceremonies should prepare one or more accords which represent one or two specific families – for example, woody/coniferous, woody/spicy, spicy/floral. These accords can be passed to the participants for examination and analysis. The odour families should be identified and recorded, the accord can be described according to its sensory characteristics, and any constituent aromatics named (this will be very difficult sometimes, depending on the number of materials used!). At the end of this exercise, the answers can be freely discussed.

Building bridges

The master of ceremonies selects between three and five aromatics, and reveals their identities to the participants; blotters should be prepared for each person. The aim of this exercise is to suggest additional aromatics that could build olfactory bridges between the selected scents. The participants should be given quiet time to assess the samples and consider their answers. The answers should be recorded and gathered by the record keeper. This can be followed by a free exchange of the ideas, and blotters with the suggested aromatic bridges can be prepared, to be smelled and compared with the selected ones. This exercise is particularly useful for broadening our perspectives on olfactory characteristics, because we will hear about individual perceptions; although we all smell the same aromatics, we will tend to pick up on or even fixate on different aspects. However, once someone remarks upon a particular note or effect, and perhaps gives a colourful description or metaphor, we too will usually 'get it'.

Scent association and inspiration

Scents have an enormous evocative impact. They may trigger a specific memory or a sensation or feeling linked to a previous experience, they might evoke a new feeling within us, and they have a vast array of associations – with images, shapes, colours, tones, sounds, words, names, notes, music, textures. This exercise allows us to explore these 'cross-modal' associations, and helps us to verbalise scent-evoked sensations.

The master of ceremonies selects three aromatics. Blotters should be prepared and, as before, are presented one at a time to the participants. The master of ceremonies can then ask a question for each scent. For example:

- If this scent was a musical instrument, or a piece of music, what would it be?

- If this scent was a season, what would it be?
- What kind of weather does this scent evoke?
- Does this scent evoke a scene in the natural world?

Each participant should record their answers, which can be collected for discussion at the end of the exercise. Following this, one scent can be chosen by each participant, who can then write a short piece about anything that this inspires. This might be a short descriptive essay, a poem, a meditation, a personal reflection, or simply a collection of phrases. There are no rules! Sometimes, a scent might not be evocative for an individual, and this is fine. Simply chose another one that 'works'.

For example, a coniferous fragrance might evoke 'a rainy autumn day in a forest', and this can be described in detail – sights, sounds, sensations. An exotic flower scent could transport the individual to a 'peaceful, lush, tropical island', and again this can be imagined and conveyed with descriptive words. Or the aromatic might conjure up feelings and sensations; for example, soft, gentle, balsamic scents might evoke feelings of being wrapped in warm fluffy blankets, while some herbal aromatics might conjure up the feeling of sunshine on the skin. Sometimes scents might evoke places where specific feelings might be experienced. Sometimes the scent can be associated with a specific memory, which can be re-experienced and described, while at other times something quite abstract and seemingly unrelated to the specific aromatic might emerge.

At the end of the exercise the answers to the questions can be discussed and the creative writing shared, if desired. Most individuals will be happy to do this, unless, of course, their words are of a private nature.

13

Reflections on the Olfactory Journey

It is often said that a journey is more important than its destination, and here this certainly holds true. The reality is that there are always more scents to explore, whether in nature, or as aromatic extracts, or in fragrances created on the way.

Fragrance can become part of us, our way of being and relating to our world. It seems fitting to reflect on Roudnitska's words!

> The more we penetrate odours, the more they end up possessing us. They live within us, becoming an integral part of us, participating in a new function within us. (Roudnitska 1991, cited by Aftel 2008, p.44)

Essentially, he is saying that the effort of exploring scents is amply rewarded by their integration in our lives; our experience is enhanced by them, and they can become part of our self-development and personal growth. He may also be referring to the development of an olfactory memory.

Scent is unchanging – when we smell fragrant plants, we smell exactly what our ancestors smelled, and we realise that scent connects the present to the past. This journey might then inspire us to explore the fascinating history of aromatics, how our ancestors experienced and were inspired or influenced by scents; or the world of perfumery; or the abundance of literature that celebrates scent. With the experience of appreciating the many exquisite scents enjoyed by mankind over the centuries, listening to scent and developing the ability to speak its language, our internal olfactory landscape becomes so very much richer; we have created a very personal, indelible, inner treasure trove.

Part II

OLFACTORY PROFILES

14

Balsamic Family

Labdanum resinoid/absolute

Botanical source

Cistus ladaniferus oleoresin (gum)

Odour profile

TYPE: balsamic, ambra (recalling ambergris – complex, rich, musty, musky, earthy and ambery)

CHARACTERISTICS: rich, sweet, soft

SUBSIDIARY NOTES AND NUANCES: woody, herbaceous

Olfactory notes

- No one component is attributable to the odour.
- Constituents include acetopheneone and its derivatives, phenols, lactones and acids. Dihydroambrinol (powerful woody-amber), α-ambrinol (strong, amber and woody, damp earth), drimenone (powerful tobacco and amber) and various other components give soft, warm, woody amber notes, sometimes with animalic or resinous variations.
- Remarkable persistence.
- A valued and important fixative in perfumery.
- Often used in base accords and part of the classic chypre fragrance base, along with oakmoss, sandalwood and musk.
- Also used as a food and beverage (alcohol and soft drinks) flavour.

Compare with

- Cistus oil: ambra, herbaceous, intense, powerful, dry/powdery, rich and warm with woody and balsamic nuances; cistus essential oil is obtained from the aerial parts of *C. ladaniferus*.

Opopanax resinoid

Botanical source

Commiphora erythraea oleogum resin

Odour profile

TYPE: balsamic, spicy

CHARACTERISTICS: fresh, warm, sweet

SUBSIDIARY NOTES AND NUANCES: floral, resinous, woody, olibanum-like (frankincense-like)

Olfactory notes

- At the 'far end' of the balsamic spectrum.
- Probably the 'myrrh' of ancient times.
- Constituents include *cis*-α-bisabolene (sweet, balsamic, spicy), α-santalene (mild, woody), and β-caryophyllene (light, spicy, clove-like, woody).
- Often used in base accords, especially in oriental fragrances.
- Sometimes called opoponax.

Compare with

- Myrrh essential oil: spicy, borderline balsamic, sharp with a medicated nuance (obtained from *C. myrrha* oleoresin and others in the genus).
- Myrrh resinoid: spicy, borderline balsamic, light, fresh, warm, less medicated than the essential oil (obtained from *C. myrrha* oleoresin and others in the genus).
- Olibanum essential oil: terpenic, lemony, woody, spicy, borderline balsamic (obtained from the oleogum resin of *Boswellia* species, mainly *B. carterii*).
- Olibanum resinoid: resinous, green, lemony, fresh, borderline balsamic (obtained from the oleogum resin of *Boswellia* species, mainly *B. carterii*).

Tolu balsam resinoid/distilled oil

Botanical source

Myroxylon toluiferum balsam

Odour profile

TYPE: balsamic, cinnamate (warm, heavy and balsamic with a fruity, strawberry-like note)

CHARACTERISTICS: warm, sweet, rich

SUBSIDIARY NOTES AND NUANCES: vanilla, hyacinth-like, spice, cinnamon

Olfactory notes

- The odour is contributed by aromatic acids (including benzoic and cinnamic acids), cinnamic alcohol (sweet, balsamic, floral, hyacinth-like and rosy), the aromatic esters benzyl benzoate (faint, sweet, balsamic) and benzyl cinnamate (mild, sweet, balsamic), and the aromatic aldehyde vanillin (4-hydroxy-3-methoxybenzaldehyde), which is intense, sweet and typical of vanilla.
- Often used in base accords and is a useful fixative.
- Imparts warmth and substance.

Compare with

- Benzoin resinoid: balsamic, sweet, soft, warm; Siam benzoin has a chocolate-like nuance, and is preferred in perfumery; Sumatra benzoin has a powdery nuance; it can contain up to 5 per cent vanillin. Benzoin has skin-sensitising potential.
- Peru balsam: balsamic, sweet, rich and soft, with vanilla, cinnamate and benzoate (pungent, floral, fruity, blackcurrant-like) nuances; the botanical source is *Myroxylon pereirae*, and the balsam is a skin sensitiser.
- Styrax: balsamic and sweet with cinnamate and naphthalene (mothball) nuances. The botanical source is the gum of *Liquidambar orientalis* or *L. styraciflua*. The gum itself is a sensitiser.
- Vanilla absolute: vanillic, balsamic, sweet, rich and warm with nuances of wood and tobacco; from the cured pods of *Vanilla planifolia*.

Vanilla absolute

Botanical source

The cured pods of *Vanilla planifolia*

Odour profile

TYPE: vanillic, balsamic

CHARACTERISTICS: sweet, rich, warm

SUBSIDIARY NOTES AND NUANCES: woody, tobacco-like

Olfactory notes

- The vanilla odour is contributed by an aromatic aldehyde called vanillin (4-hydroxy-3-methoxybenzaldehyde), which crystallises on the surface of cured vanilla pods; in the absolute it is present at around 2 per cent; vanillin itself has an intense, sweet vanilla odour; both naturally derived and synthetic vanillins are used in perfumery.
- Often used in base accords and is a good fixative.
- Often used as a tobacco aroma/flavour.
- Imparts sweet, soft, smooth qualities.

Compare with

- Benzoin resinoid: balsamic, sweet, soft, warm; Siam benzoin has a chocolate-like nuance, and is preferred in perfumery; Sumatra benzoin has a powdery nuance; it can contain up to 5 per cent vanillin. The botanical source is the resin of *Styrax tonkinensis* (Siam). Overuse in a formula has the effect of deadening or suppressing other aromatics; benzoin has skin-sensitising potential.
- Cacao absolute: balsamic, rich and warm, with chocolate nuances, but vanilla is absent; the botanical source is *Theobroma cacao* seeds.
- Peru balsam: balsamic, sweet, rich and soft, with vanilla, cinnamate (warm, heavy and balsamic with a fruity strawberry-like note) and benzoate (pungent, floral, fruity, blackcurrant-like) nuances; the botanical source is *Myroxylon pereirae* balsam, and the non-distilled balsam is a known skin sensitiser.
- Tolu balsam: balsamic, sweet, with cinnamate and vanillic nuances; the botanical source is *Myroxylon toluiferum* balsam.

Balsamic Family

15

Woody Family

Guaiacwood essential oil

Botanical source

Bulnesia sarmientoi wood

Odour profile

TYPE: woody

CHARACTERISTICS: soft, sweet, clean

SUBSIDIARY NOTES AND NUANCES: tea rose, balsamic

Olfactory notes

- Sometimes called champaca wood oil; the wood contains guaiac resin which causes a blue-green discoloration in cut wood.
- Essential oil is crystalline, melting at 45°C.
- Contains guaiol and guaiene (smoky, powerful, medicated), guiayl acetate (woody, balsamic, vetiver-like) and guaiacwood acetate (soft, sweet, warm, rosy, woody).
- Functions as a base–middle note and has fixative qualities.
- Some oils might have a smoky nuance.
- Guaiacwood acetate is a sweet, delicate, woody-rosy derivative of the oil, and is used in rose and violet compositions.

Compare with

- Rosewood essential oil: woody, floral (rosy); look for the slightly camphoraceous top note; fresh, with spicy nuances. The botanical source is *Aniba rosaeodora*.

East Indian sandalwood essential oil

Botanical source

Santalum album heartwood and roots

Odour profile

TYPE: woody

CHARACTERISTICS: soft, sweet

SUBSIDIARY NOTES AND NUANCES: balsamic, fatty, animalic, milky, musky, urinous

Olfactory notes

- Lacks a top note.
- Very persistent base note and a good fixative.
- Some individuals can detect a urinous note.
- Dominant constituents are α- and β-santalols; the α-santalols confer woody, cedar-like attributes; the warm-woody, milky, musky, urinous and animalic characteristics are contributed mainly by the β-santalols and traces of 2-α-*trans*-bergamotol, a sesquiterpenoid; the constituent responsible for the tenacity is β-santalene.
- A few individuals experience partial anosmia with sandalwood.

Compare with

- *S. spicatum* essential oil: soft, woody, extremely tenacious, balsamic, sweet, with a dry, spicy, resinous top note.
- *S. austrocaledonicum* essential oil: woody, sandalwood-like, amber nuances, less resinous than *S. spicatum*.

Woody Family

Virginian cedarwood essential oil

Botanical source

Juniperus virginiana wood

Odour profile

TYPE: woody

CHARACTERISTICS: mild, dry, light, fresh

SUBSIDIARY NOTES AND NUANCES: woody/oily, resinous, balsamic, earthy

Olfactory notes

- Obtained from the 'eastern red cedar', but is actually a species of juniper.
- Look for the 'pencil shavings' nuance.
- Dominant constituents are α-cedrol (woody, cedar-like); α- and β-cedrene (woody cedar, slightly camphoraceous); thujopsene (cedar-like); β-caryophyllene (light, spicy, clove-like, woody) and γ-eudesmol (sweet, woody).
- Often used as a reference for the woody odour type.
- Used in top note accords, to impart woody effects.
- Has fixative properties.

Compare with

- Hibawood essential oil: woody, intense, pungent; from *Thujopsis dolobrata*.
- Atlas cedarwood essential oil: woody, slightly oily, warm, slightly camphoraceous; from *Cedrus atlantica*.
- Himalayan cedarwood essential oil: woody, with sweet, resinous and urinous notes, and, in unrectified oil, a 'dirty', slightly crude note; rectified oils which have a more pleasant odour are preferred; from *C. deodara*.
- Chinese cedar: sweet, woody, with a 'pencil shavings' nuance; from a species of cypress, *Cupressus funebris*.
- Juniperberry essential oil: terpenic, coniferous (pine-like), resinous, woody, balsamic, fresh; from berries of *Juniperus communis*; the terpenic odour type falls in the medicated family.

16

Spicy Family

Caraway seed essential oil (normally rectified)

Botanical source

Carum carvi dried seeds

Odour profile

TYPE: spicy

CHARACTERISTICS: very intense, warm, sweet

SUBSIDIARY NOTES AND NUANCES: weedy (in top note)

Olfactory notes

- The essential oil is usually rectified.
- Odour is very similar to dried, crushed seeds.
- Dominant constituent is *d*-carvone which has the odour of caraway, while the molecule's mirror image, *l*-carvone, smells minty. (See also peppermint, comparison with spearmint.)
- Very intense, so used sparingly.
- In perfumery, is used to complement jasmine or cassie absolute (from *Acacia farnesiana*), and in tabac and fougère fragrances.
- Used as a 'mask' in insecticides and to flavour mouthwashes.

Compare with

- Carrot seed essential oil: spicy, woody, earthy, fresh and sweet; the botanical source is the dried seeds of *Daucus carota*.
- Celery seed essential oil: spicy, diffusive, rich and warm; the botanical source is the crushed seeds of *Apium graveolens*.
- Coriander seed essential oil: fresh, sweet, spicy and woody, with floral and citrus nuances; the botanical source is the dried, fully ripe seeds of *Coriandrum sativum*.
- Cumin seed essential oil: distinctive, spicy, earthy, warm, powerful, with 'unwashed sweaty body odour' nuances; the botanical source is *Cuminum cyminum* (dried seeds).
- Fenugreek essential oil: intense, woody, spicy, warm, rich, with initial curry-like and then walnut-like nuances; the fresh, crushed seeds have a celery-like odour. The botanical source is *Trigonella foenum-graecum* (seeds).

Carrot seed essential oil

Botanical source

Daucus carota dried seeds

Odour profile

TYPE: spicy

CHARACTERISTICS: fresh, sweet, persistent

SUBSIDIARY NOTES AND NUANCES: earthy, rooty, woody

Olfactory notes

- Quite intense and persistent, so used sparingly.

- Dominant constituents are the sesquiterpene alcohols carotol and daucol, also α- and β-pinene (fresh, pine-like), geraniol (rosy), geranyl acetate (sweet, rosy and fruity), *l*-limonene (weak citrus), caryophyllene (woody and spicy, clove-like) and others.

- In perfumery, carrot seed oil is used in the top notes of 'natural type' fragrances, fougères and chypres.

- The combination of carrot seed and cedarwood can mimic the scent of orris oil (concrete), a valued fragrance material obtained from the dried rhizomes of *Iris pallida, I. germanica* and *I. florentina*. In order to allow the fragrance to develop, the rhizomes must be washed, peeled and then dried under controlled conditions for three years.

Compare with

- Coriander seed essential oil: fresh, sweet, spicy, peppery and woody, with floral and citrus nuances; the botanical source is the dried, fully ripe seeds of *Coriandrum sativum*.

- Sweet fennel essential oil: fresh, sweet, spicy, anisic and earthy; the botanical source is the dried seeds of *Foeniculum vulgare* var. *dulce*.

- Black pepper essential oil: fresh, dry, spicy and woody; the botanical source is the dried, crushed, almost ripe seeds of *Piper nigrum*. Although this is fresh, it is not sweet, and note just how different this makes the odour when compared with the others in the spicy category; a peppery note can be found in coriander seed (above) and also bergamot (see the citrus family).

- Nutmeg essential oil: fresh, spicy and warm, but with pine-like nuances; from the nutmeg seed, *Myristica fragrans*.

Spicy Family

Clove bud essential oil

Botanical source

Syzygium aromaticum dried unopened flower buds

Odour profile

TYPE: spicy

CHARACTERISTICS: rich, warm, sweet

SUBSIDIARY NOTES AND NUANCES: fruity, woody

Olfactory notes

- Clove bud essential oil has a scent directly related to the spice, but make a comparison with the crushed, dried cloves.
- In perfumery it is used in very small amounts, but adds spicy warmth to fragrances, especially rose and carnation types.
- The dominant constituent is eugenol, which is warm, spicy and clove-like; eugenol can be used as a raw material for the synthesis of vanillin (see the balsamic family).

Compare with

- Cassia essential oil (rectified): sweet, warm and spicy with cinnamon-like nuances; the botanical source is the inner bark of *Cinnamomum cassia*.
- Cinnamon leaf essential oil: harsh, pungent, warm and spicy odour, typical of cinnamon, but also reminiscent of clove, with sweet fruity nuances; the botanical source is the dried leaves of *Cinnamomum camphorum*.
- Cinnamon bark essential oil: strong, sweet, warm, fruity and spicy, with powdery, floral and clove nuances; it is preferred over the leaf oil in perfumery. The botanical source is the dried inner bark of *Cinnamomum camphorum*.
- Pimento essential oil: fresh, sweet, warm and spicy, with tea-like (see also clary sage of the herbaceous family), clove and nutmeg nuances; the botanical source is the dried unripe berries of *Pimento dioica*.
- West Indian bay essential oil: fresh, spicy and sweet, and dominated by eugenol – look for the clove-like effect. Obtained from the leaves of *Pimenta racemosa*.

Spicy Family

Nutmeg essential oil

Botanical source

Myristica fragrans fruit kernels

Odour profile

TYPE: spicy

CHARACTERISTICS: fresh, warm

SUBSIDIARY NOTES AND NUANCES: sweet, pine-like, ethereal

Olfactory notes

- Compare the essential oil with the freshly ground spice.
- Nutmeg oil is dominated by a group of constituents known as monoterpenes (such as camphene, α- and β-pinene, which have fresh, piney, penetrating odours), monoterpene alcohols (such as the floral and lilac-like α-terpineol; the camphoraceous and woody borneol; the rosy geraniol and the mild, soft floral/woody linalool); and the clove-like phenol in its two forms, eugenol and *iso*-eugenol. However, it also contains the aromatic (phenolic) ether myristicin, or methoxysafrole, which is important in the nutmeg aroma; it is sweet, warm and spicy.
- Myristicin has also been found in members of the carrot family.
- In perfumery the 'East Indian' oil from Indonesia and Sri Lanka is preferred over the 'West Indian' oil from Grenada.
- Nutmeg is also used to flavour tobacco products.

Compare with

- Mace essential oil: very similar to nutmeg, but less pine-like in the top notes; obtained from the 'aril', the red husk that surrounds the nutmeg.
- Pimento essential oil: fresh, sweet, warm and spicy, with clove and nutmeg nuances; the botanical source is the dried, unripe berries of *Pimento dioica*.
- Sweet fennel essential oil: fresh, sweet, anisic and earthy; look for the ethereal note provided by a phenolic (aromatic) ether called *trans*-anethole. The botanical source is the dried seeds of *Foeniculum vulgare* var. *dulce*.
- Clove bud essential oil: rich, warm and spicy, but with fruity and woody nuances; obtained from the unopened flower buds of *Syzygium aromaticum*.
- Bay laurel essential oil: fresh, warm, spicy, sweet and slightly clove-like, with camphoraceous nuances; obtained from the leaves of *Laurus nobilis*. The absolute (see laurel leaf in the herbaceous family) is preferred in perfumery.

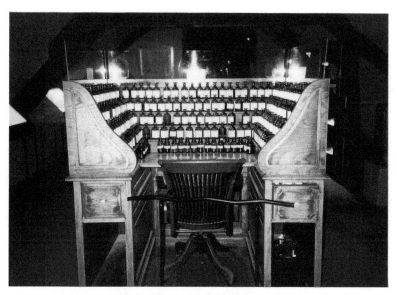

Colour Plate 1 The perfumer's organ
This traditional perfumer's organ can be seen at the Château de Chamerolles in France, which is now dedicated to the history of fragrances and the art of perfume – *La Promenade des Parfums*.
Image: Derek Rhind

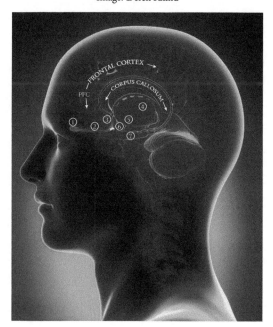

Colour Plate 2 The human olfactory system
1. Olfactory bulb; 2. Olfactory nerve; 3. Olfactory pathway; 4. Region of thalamus (relay system for signals between nervous system and brain); 5. Region of hypothalamus (monitors and maintains bodily functions); 6. Region of amygdala (basic emotions); 7. Region of hippocampus (memory):
Frontal cortex (organising and planning); PFC: prefrontal cortex (executive, logical, social decisions).
Image: Shutterstock

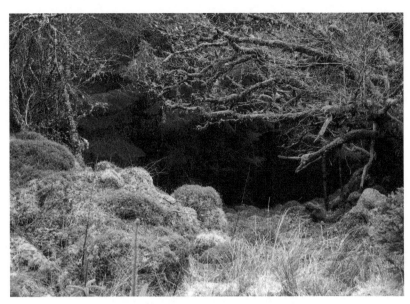

Colour Plate 3 Shinrin-yoku – a coniferous forest
This is the walk through a largely coniferous forest on the way to the remote beach at
Gortenfern, Kentra Bay – or the 'Singing Sands', Ardnamurchan. The air was filled
with the scents of conifers, and the salty tang of sea air became stronger as Kentra Bay
was reached. (See www.moidart.com/walking-ardnamurchan/singing-sands.)
Image: Derek Rhind

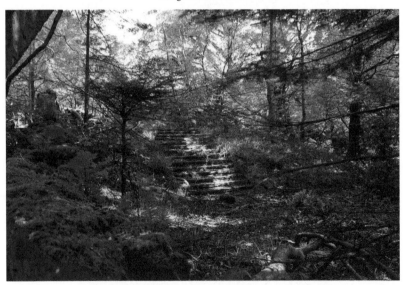

Colour Plate 4 Shinrin-yoku – a deciduous wood
Providing a contrast to the environment and scents of a coniferous forest, this mixed broadleaf
deciduous woodland borders Saddle Bay, Kintryre. The scents were beautiful, green and earthy.
The bluebells did not have a perfume, but they certainly added to the special atmosphere.
Image: Derek Rhind

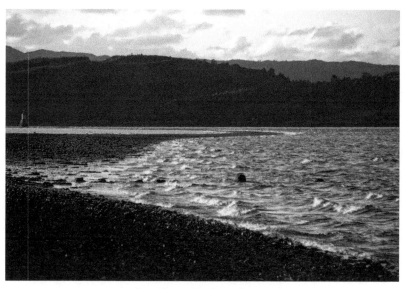

Colour Plate 5 The shore of a sea loch

There is nothing quite like the atmosphere of the Scottish sea loch! This is at Otter Ferry, on Loch Fyne, Argyll, and shows the long seaweed-covered spit that reaches way across the loch. The air was fresh and bracing, and we could certainly smell fresh seaweed too. The fishy smell of decay was completely absent. (See www.argyllsecretcoast.co.uk/viewdetails.php?id=128&rf=secret-magical-spots.)

Image: Derek Rhind

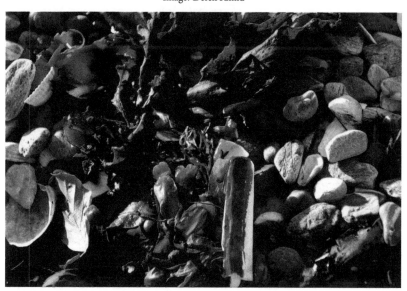

Colour Plate 6 Close-up of the beach

Compare this with Colour Plate 5 – can you imagine the difference in odour? This is at Mellon Udrigle – a stunning beach with views across to mountains and the Summer Isles, in Wester Ross. The close-up lets us see shells, pebbles and different types of seaweed. Here, the air had a fresh, briny quality, and the shore itself smelled of seaweed and salt; it was quite intense, but fresh and pleasant. (See www.visitscotland.com/info/towns-villages/mellon-udrigle-beach-p730881.)

Image: Derek Rhind

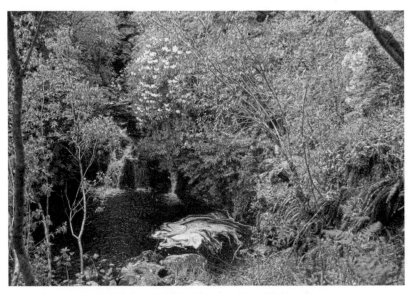

Colour Plate 7 A Himalayan-style woodland garden

In late spring, the stunning Crarae Garden at Minard, near Inveraray on Loch Fyne, Argyll, is filled with the heady scents of Rhododendron species, including the intense, pervasive perfume of the yellow blossoms of *R. luteum*. Although visually impressive, and lovely at any time of year, if you visit when the rhododendrons are in flower, the experience is immensely enhanced by their scents. (See www.gardens-of-argyll.co.uk/gardens/crarae-garden.html.)

Image: Derek Rhind

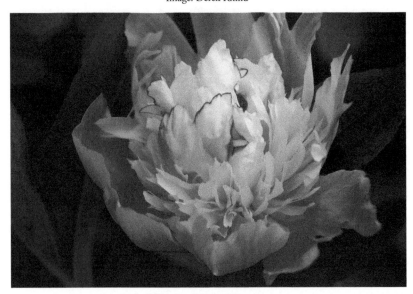

Colour Plate 8 Peony blossom

This close-up of a peony blossom gives a dramatic example of how our senses of sight and smell are linked by association. Here, Paeonia lactiflora 'Sorbet' has a pink centre of petals edged with a deeper raspberry shade, and pink guard petals, separated by a ruff of cream petals. This flower is reminiscent of a vanilla and raspberry dessert, perhaps ice cream, and the scent is indeed sweet, and recalls this!

Image: Derek Rhind

17

Coniferous Family

Scots pine essential oil

Botanical source

Pinus sylvestris leaves (needles), twigs and cones

Odour profile

TYPE: coniferous, pine

CHARACTERISTICS: fresh, harsh, strong

SUBSIDIARY NOTES AND NUANCES: woody, resinous, balsamic, terpenic, turpentine

Olfactory notes

- Represents the pine sub-family.
- Also called the Norway pine.
- Dominated by monoterpenes, notably α- and β-pinene (resinous and woody) and δ-3-carene (sweet, harsh and lemony); also *l*-limonene (weak, mint-like), myrcene (sweet and balsamic), ocimene (light and herbaceous) and other monoterpenes; the ester bornyl acetate (camphoraceous and pine-like) and the oxide 1,8-cineole (eucalyptus-like).
- Pine oils and the pinenes have acquired associations with household disinfectant products because of their extensive use in this category.
- Inhalation of pine oil can relieve bronchial and sinus congestion.

Compare with

- Dwarf pine essential oil: sweet, woody and balsamic, and more tenacious than other pine oils; sometimes described as 'unique' and preferred in perfumery, but not in aromatherapy because it is an irritant and sensitiser. The oil is characterised by the presence of lower aliphatic (short chain) aldehydes and cyclic aldehydes. Botanical sources are the young shoots and needles of *Pinus mugo* var. *pumilio*, and *P. montana*.
- Longleaf pine essential oil: fresh, coniferous, pine, terpenic and turpentine-like and disinfectant-like. The botanical source is the needles and twigs of *Pinus palustris*, which is also the source of turpentine, distilled from the oleoresin that exudes from the trunk.

Siberian fir essential oil

Botanical source

Abies sibirica young shoots and needles

Odour profile

TYPE: coniferous, pine

CHARACTERISTICS: fresh, sweet

SUBSIDIARY NOTES AND NUANCES: balsamic, fruity (citrus)

Olfactory notes

* Representative of the pine sub-family.
* Generally, fir oils have fresh, typically coniferous scents, sometimes with a lemony aspect, and often lack the resinous base notes of the pines and junipers. Typical constituents are α- and β-pinene (resinous and woody), myrcene (sweet and balsamic), δ-3-carene (sweet, harsh and lemony), bornyl acetate (camphoraceous and pine-like), *d*- (weak lemony) and *l*-limonene (turpentine, minty), and phellandrene (fresh, lemony, woody).
* Used as a top note in perfumery.
* Many species are used to produce so-called 'fir' essential oils, including species of *Larix* (larch), *Picea* (spruce) and *Tsuga* (hemlock).

Compare with

* Balsam fir essential oil and absolute: also known as the Canadian balsam fir (*A. balsamea*); the absolute has a very pronounced coniferous, forest scent with a sweet, fruity nuance. This tree also yields an oleoresin called Canada balsam – regarded as an excellent fixative, which can be steam distilled to yield an essential oil with a sweet balsamic and pine-like odour.
* Grand fir essential oil: look for the orange-like nuance; obtained from *A. grandis*.
* Silver fir essential oil: sweet, rich, with a balsamic character; obtained from *A. alba* needles and twigs and sometimes cones.
* *A. sachalinensis* essential oil: also typical of the fir type.
* Spruce essential oils: less readily available in some countries, but can be obtained from the black spruce (*Picea mariana*), the white spruce (*P. alba*), the Norway spruce (*P. abies*), the Canadian white spruce (*P. canadensis*) and the Icelandic red spruce (*P. rubens*).

Coniferous Family

18
Herbaceous Family

Clary sage essential oil

Botanical source

Salvia sclarea flowering tops and leaves

Odour profile

TYPE: herbal

CHARACTERISTICS: sweet, light, warm

SUBSIDIARY NOTES AND NUANCES: tobacco-like, tea-like, hay, woody/cedar, balsamic

Olfactory notes

- Very distinctive odour.
- The dominant constituents are similar to lavender: linalool (mild, floral, woody) and linalyl acetate (sweet, floral, fruity, bergamot-like); however, clary is complex, and contains over 250 constituents, including an unusual diterpene alcohol named sclareol.
- Sclareol has a delicate, ambergris-like odour.
- Clary oil and absolute are widely used in the flavour and fragrance industries.

Compare with

- Sage essential oil: often said to be a typical representative of the herbaceous family, sage oil is warm, herbal, camphoraceous – sometimes with urinous nuances. It has a very different chemical make-up, being dominated by ketones that are associated with neurotoxicity, notably α- and β-thujone, and camphor (perhaps wise to avoid in epilepsy). The botanical source is *S. officinalis*; it is sometimes called Dalmatian sage.
- East Mediterranean (or Greek or Cretan) sage essential oil: herbal with camphoraceous and eucalyptus-like nuances; the botanical source is *S. libanotica*.
- Spanish (or lavender-leaved) sage essential oil: fresh, herbal, with camphoraceous, eucalyptus-like and pine-like nuances; the botanical source is *S. lavandulaefolia*.
- Artemisia essential oil: sweet, fresh, herbal, with warm, camphoraceous and woody nuances; the botanical source is the aerial parts of *Artemisia herba-alba*. There are several chemotypes; it contains α- and β-thujone, camphor and 1,8-cineole, and also 'artemisia alcohol'. In perfumery this odour type is defined as 'armoise'; the absolute is also worth exploring.
- Clary sage absolute: sweet, light, warm and subtle, herbal and persistent, with woody and ambra nuances.

Laurel leaf absolute

Botanical source

Laurus nobilis leaves

Odour profile

TYPE: herbal

CHARACTERISTICS: fresh, warm, aromatic

SUBSIDIARY NOTES AND NUANCES: green, spicy

Olfactory notes

- Sometimes called bay laurel.
- Bay laurel essential oil is better known than the absolute; however, it has been implicated in contact allergic reactions causing redness and severe inflammation. It is dominated by 1,8-cineole (eucalyptus-like), with other monoterpene derivatives and traces of a toxic phenolic ether: methyl eugenol (which is sweet, herbaceous and anisic).
- Laurel leaf absolute is preferred in perfumery, although its use is restricted.
- In perfumery the absolute is used in aromatic and fresh fougère fragrance types as well as spicy oriental fragrances.

Compare with

- Bay laurel essential oil: similar to the leaves, with fresh, sweet herbal, spicy, clove-like nuances, but also camphoraceous and cineolic notes which are not present in the absolute.
- Nutmeg essential oil: fresh, spicy and warm, with pine-like nuances; look for the sweet, ethereal notes given by its aromatic ether, myristicin (obtained from the nutmeg seed, *Myristica fragrans*).
- Basil essential oil (exotic, methyl chavicol chemotype): fresh herbal; look for the sweet, anisic nuances given by its aromatic ether methyl chavicol (also known as 'estragole'). The botanical source is *Ocimum basilicum* leaves.
- Tulsi (holy basil) essential oil: aromatic, sweet and herbaceous, with clove-like nuances, partly due to the presence of eugenol and estragole, depending on the variety; some varieties have a characteristic cassis (blackcurrant bud) note. The botanical source is *Ocimum sanctum*.
- Sweet fennel essential oil: fresh, sweet, anisic and earthy; also look for the ethereal note provided by an aromatic ether called *trans*-anethole. The botanical source is the dried seeds of *Foeniculum vulgare* var. *dulce*.

True lavender essential oil

Botanical source

Lavandula angustifolia (*L. officinalis* or *L. vera*); sub-species include *delphinensis* and *fragrans*, flowering tops

Odour profile

TYPE: herbal, lavender

CHARACTERISTICS: sweet, fresh, light

SUBSIDIARY NOTES AND NUANCES: floral, fruity, woody

Olfactory notes

* Lavender essential oil from France, sold as '40/42' is typical; the '40/42' refers to its ester (linalyl acetate) content.
* Lavender essential oil is characterised by two constituents: the monoterpene alcohol *l*-linalool (mild, sweet, light, floral, woody, citrus nuances) and the ester linalyl acetate (fresh, light, herbal and bergamot-like); many others are present.
* The English oil is held in high regard; it has a lower ester content, and a higher 1,8-cineole (an oxide with a eucalyptus-like odour) content.
* Extensively used in both perfumery and aromatherapy.

Compare with

* High-altitude French lavender (50/52): look for its distinctive fruity 'pear drops' nuance.
* French lavender: more camphoraceous than true lavender; the essential oil is obtained from *L. stoechas*, and is known in the essential oil trade as 'French lavender'.
* Spike lavender essential oil: lavender-like and penetrating, but camphoraceous and lacking the soft, fruity nuances of true lavender. It contains more 1,8-cineole than lavender, and also camphor. The botanical source is *L. latifolia*, also known as *L. spica*, and it has a sub-species named *fragrans*.
* Lavandin essential oil: lavender-like; more penetrating and fresher, but less fruity than true lavender, and less camphoraceous than spike; the botanical source is the hybrid *Lavandula × intermedia*, a cross between true lavender and spike lavender.
* Lavender absolute: the odour is very similar to the plant, although more intense, sweet and herbaceous, with green, floral and hay-like nuances (from *L. angustifolia*).

White thyme (rectified) essential oil

Botanical source

Thymus vulgaris flowering tops and leaves

Odour profile

TYPE: herbal, medicated (thymolic)

CHARACTERISTICS: sharp, warm, penetrating

SUBSIDIARY NOTES AND NUANCES: woody, spicy, tobacco-like

Olfactory notes

- The first distillate is red in colour and cloudy in appearance, and this is called 'red thyme oil', which is then filtered and re-distilled to produce 'white thyme oil'; this has a sweeter top note.

- Dominated by a phenol known as thymol (powerful, medicated and herbaceous), also carvacrol (tar-like), and terpenes such as *para*-cymene (fresh, citrus, herbal), α-terpinene (lemony), camphene (mild, oily, camphoraceous) and others, such as linalool (mild, woody, floral) and geraniol (sweet, rosy, floral).

- There are several cultivated varieties, which give rise to 'chemotypes' (essential oils with differing chemistry): thymol, carvacrol, linalool and geraniol, named after their dominant constituents.

- As its odour would suggest, thyme oils are useful antimicrobials, but the thymol and carvacrol chemotypes are also skin irritants.

Compare with

- *T. vulgaris* chemotype linalool essential oil: herbal, thyme with a softer, sweeter, woodier odour.

- *T. vulgaris* chemotype geraniol essential oil: herbal, thyme with a sweeter odour and rosy nuances.

- Wild thyme (*T. serpyllum*), Moroccan thyme (*T. saturoides*), Spanish thyme (*T. zygis*), Spanish oreganum (*T. capitatus*) and Spanish marjoram (*T. mastichina*) essential oils: all with the distinctive thyme signature, but with varying nuances.

- Thyme absolute: sweet, light, warm and subtle, herbal and persistent, with woody and ambra nuances (from *T. vulgaris*).

Herbaceous Family

19

Medicated Family

Eucalyptus 'blue gum' essential oil

Botanical source

Eucalyptus globulus var. *globulus* leaves and twigs

Odour profile

TYPE: medicinal, cineolic

CHARACTERISTICS: powerful, fresh, penetrating

SUBSIDIARY NOTES AND NUANCES: camphoraceous, green

Olfactory notes

- There are three main groups of eucalyptus oils, based on their chemical composition – medicinal, industrial and perfumery (non-cineole). The 'medicinal' oils, or 'eucapharma' oils, contain significant amounts of 1,8-cineole, an oxide that has expectorant properties and can also improve blood flow to the brain. Most eucalyptus oils are rectified.

- The constituent 1,8-cineole is also known as 'eucalyptol'; its name has given rise to a specific odour type, 'cineolic' meaning 'eucalyptus-like'. Other notable constituents are monoterpenes such as α-pinene (pine-like and resinous) and *d*-limonene (weak citrus).

Compare with

- Blue-leaved mallee (*E. polybractea*) essential oil: sweet, fresh and cineolic with camphoraceous nuances; also *p*-cymene (fresh, citrus-like, herbaceous nuances), terpinen-4-ol (mild, peppery), α- and β-pinene (pine-like), *d*-limonene (weak citrus/lemony) and sabinene (warm, woody, spicy, herbaceous).

- Green mallee (*E. viridis*) essential oil: sweet, fresh and cineolic; very similar to the blue gum oil.

- Gully-gum or Smith's gum (*E. smithii*) essential oil: fresh and cineolic; also contains substantial amounts of phellandrene (fresh, mild citrus, woody, slightly spicy).

- White camphor essential oil: clean, fleeting and typical of the camphoraceous odour type that is present in many essential oils, including the cineole-rich eucalyptus ones. The botanical source is the wood of *Cinnamomum camphora*, and white camphor is the first fraction of the distillation process; it is dominated by 1,8-cineole.

- Cajuput essential oil: strong, sweet and camphoraceous; also dominated by 1,8-cineole and so has a eucalyptus nuance; from the 'paperbark' tree *Melaleuca cajuputi*.

Peppermint essential oil

Botanical source

Mentha × *piperita* leaves and twigs; a hybrid: between spearmint (*M. spicatum*) and watermint (*M. aquatica*)

Odour profile

TYPE: medicinal, mentholic

CHARACTERISTICS: strong, fresh, penetrating

SUBSIDIARY NOTES AND NUANCES: green, herbaceous

Olfactory notes

- *l*-menthol (fresh, pungent, cooling, minty) is the main constituent, along with *l*-menthone (fresh, refreshing and minty with woody nuances); also menthyl acetate (mild, sweet, herbaceous-minty nuances) and menthyl *iso*-valerate (sweet, herbaceous, minty, rooty nuances).

- Imparts a 'cooling' sensation, compared to the camphoraceous odour type, which is 'warming'; related to stimulation of the trigeminal nerve.

Compare with

- Spearmint essential oil: also 'cooling', sweet, warm, minty, green with herbaceous nuances (from *M. spicatum*, sometimes known as *M. viridis*). Its main chemical constituent is *l*-carvone (minty). Also compare with caraway essential oil (see the spicy family), which contains *d*-carvone, the optical isomer with a caraway odour.

- Pennyroyal essential oil: intense, pungent and minty with herbaceous nuances (given by main constituents pulegone, *iso*-pulegone and piperitol) and eucalyptus-like notes (1,8-cineole), spicy, thyme-like (from carvacrol) and lemon (limonene and the aldehydes octanal and nonanal) nuances; from *M. pulegium*.

- Broad-leaved peppermint (*Eucalyptus dives*) essential oil: piperitone-rich varieties have a fresh, camphoraceous, minty odour. Piperitone is an 'industrial' eucalyptus oil used in the production of menthol and thymol.

- Narrow-leaved or black peppermint (*E. radiata*) essential oil: phellandrene-rich varieties have a penetrating, peppery-camphoraceous, minty odour. Phellandrene (fresh, citrus, woody and spicy) is used in the manufacture of disinfectants and antiseptics (another 'industrial' oil).

- Mint absolute: fresh, soft, minty, green, without sharpness or harshness; from *M. piperita*.

Medicated Family

Wintergreen essential oil

Botanical source

Gaultheria procumbens leaves, treated by warm aqueous maceration

Odour profile

TYPE: medicinal, wintergreen

CHARACTERISTICS: strong, intense, sweet, penetrating

SUBSIDIARY NOTES AND NUANCES: woody, fruity

Olfactory notes

- The main constituent, an ester called methyl salicylate, is responsible for the characteristic and distinctive odour.
- Methyl salicylate itself has a sweet, medicated and fruity odour.
- Methyl salicylate is an irritant and sensitiser.
- Wintergreen oil and methyl salicylate are ingredients in traditional pharmaceuticals such as the decongestant 'Olbas oil' and pain-relieving counter-irritants.
- Wintergreen is also used in the flavour industry for personal care products (toothpastes), confectionery and soft drinks.

Compare with

- Sweet birch essential oil: intense, sweet, medicated, wintergreen with woody nuances; very similar to that of wintergreen. From the warm aqueous macerated bark of *Betula lenta*.
- Ylang ylang extra essential oil: sweet, persistent, diffusive and floral, with a fruity character and creamy nuances. Look for the medicated note imparted by methyl salicylate. The botanical source is *Cananga odorata* var. *genuina* flowers.
- Frangipani (*Plumeria rubra* varieties) absolute: sweet, tea-rose-like, with spicy-herbaceous notes; methyl salicylate is present in some varieties and may (along with other constituents) contribute to the sweet, spicy/herbaceous/fruity nuances.

20
Green Family

Violet leaf absolute

Botanical source

Viola odorata leaves

Odour profile

TYPE: green

CHARACTERISTICS: intense, diffusive, sharp

SUBSIDIARY NOTES AND NUANCES: leafy (crushed green leaves), peppery, floral/violet, woody, earthy

Olfactory notes

- The chemical composition of violet leaf is complex; however, the component that is responsible for the distinctive odour is 2-trans-6-*cis*-nonadien-1-al.
- Violet leaf is used, in small doses, to give natural green effects in the middle notes of fragrances.
- It is often used in rose bases.
- Best experienced in dilution – the odour of the absolute has been described as unpleasant because of its intensity.
- Can also be considered in a green sub-family in the context of the agrestic family.

Compare with

- Shiso mint essential oil: fresh, green, peppery, with nuances of apple seed, basil, cumin and caraway. Shiso is an Asian mint (*Perilla frutescens, P. nankin*) that is better known in cuisine but coming to the fore in perfumery.
- Blackcurrant bud absolute: illustrates a very different context for the green odour type; intense, powerful, diffusive, green, fruity, minty and 'catty'; in perfumery it is sometimes used to modify intense green notes. From *Ribes nigrum* flower buds.
- Tagetes essential oil: again, the green odour type in a fruity but herbaceous context; this is warm, sweet, fruity, apple-like and green-herbaceous. From the aerial parts of *Tagetes glandulifera*.
- Tarragon essential oil: very different in character, here the green odour type is experienced in a sweet, anisic, powdery context. Compare also with basil and artemisia (*A. herba-alba*) oils to get a sense of the close relationship between green, anisic, herbaceous and armoise odour types. Obtained from *Artemisia dracunculus*.

Galbanum essential oil

Botanical source

Ferula galbaniflua oleoresin

Odour profile

TYPE: green

CHARACTERISTICS: intense, fresh, sharp

SUBSIDIARY NOTES AND NUANCES: cut green bell peppers, coniferous, pine-like, old wood, earthy, musty

Olfactory notes

- The component responsible for the distinctive odour is the nitrogen-containing pyrazine called 2-methoxy-3-*iso*-butylpyrazine and undecatriene-3-one; however, it is dominated by monoterpenes including the pinenes (notably β-pinene), which accounts for the piney characteristics, δ-3-carene (sweet, harsh and lemony) and *l*-limonene.
- Galbanum oil is used, in small doses, to give natural green effects in the top notes of fragrances.
- It is often used in chypre and fougère fragrance types, also in hyacinth, narcissus and gardenia fragrances.
- In perfumery, 'galbanol', a deterpenated product, is sometimes used; this does not have the strong piney nuances.
- Best experienced in 10 per cent dilution – the odour of the absolute has been described as unpleasant because of its intensity.
- Can also be considered in a green sub-family in the context of the agrestic family.

Compare with

- Galbanum resinoid: sharp, green, coniferous, but with balsamic notes and more pronounced earthy nuances than the oil; used as a base note and fixative in green, floral, chypre and fougère fragrances.

21

Agrestic Family

Hay absolute

Botanical source

Hierochloe alpina dried grass

Odour profile

TYPE: agrestic

CHARACTERISTICS: rich, warm, sweet

SUBSIDIARY NOTES AND NUANCES: green, hay-like

Olfactory notes

- *H. alpina* is also known as alpine sweetgrass, and is related to the sweetgrass (*H. odorata*) that is used in Native American ceremonies and rituals.

- Hay absolute is used occasionally in perfumery, but more often the cheaper synthetic coumarin (new-mown hay odour) is used.

- Coumarin occurs naturally in tonka bean and melilot (*Melilotus officinalis* or sweet clover) and in smaller amounts in lavender and narcissus.

- Coumarin is important in the fougère fragrance type, but can also be found in chypre, lavender and herbal fragrances.

- The cut grass (*foin coupé*) type of fragrance can be reproduced by combining synthetic coumarin with deterpenated bergamot and lavender, and then synthetic methyl salicylate (which has a wintergreen odour), clary sage and oakmoss.

Compare with

- Flouve essential oil: sweet, hay with vanilla nuances, mimosa-like, imparted by coumarin and benzoic acid. The absolute is called *foin*. The botanical source is the sweet-scented vernal grass (*Anthoxanthum odoratum*).

- Tonka bean absolute: rich, sweet, warm, subtle, hay-like with herbaceous, vanillic and coconut-like nuances; used as a fixative. The botanical source is *Dipteryx odorata* beans.

- Lavender absolute: the odour that is very similar to the plant, although more intense, sweet and herbaceous, with green, floral and hay-like nuances (from *Lavandula angustifolia*).

- Narcissus absolute: heavy, sweet, herbaceous, hay-like, earthy, floral odour; it only smells like narcissus on extreme dilution. The botanical source is *Narcissus poeticus*.

Oakmoss absolute

Botanical source

Evernia prunastri lichen

Odour profile

TYPE: agrestic, mossy

CHARACTERISTICS: smooth, rich, warm, sweet

SUBSIDIARY NOTES AND NUANCES: earthy, woody, resinous, honey-like, hay-like

Olfactory notes

- Oakmoss has been used in perfumery for thousands of years, for its fragrance and outstanding fixative properties.
- Very important in the chypre type of fragrance, where it is combined with labdanum, sandalwood and musk to provide the base note (patchouli and clary sage are often included too), with a floral (rose and jasmine) heart, and top notes of bergamot and other citrus oils.
- It is complex, and contains unusual esters such as ethyl evernate, ethyl divaricatinate, ethyl haematommate, methyl-β-orcinol carboxylate, ethers such as orcinyl monomethylether, and some more familiar constituents such as borneol (camphoraceous, woody), bornyl acetate (camphoraceous, pine-like), linalool (mild, woody, floral) and 1,8-cineole (eucalyptus-like).
- Some of the constituents of oakmoss have the potential to cause sensitisation and cross-reactivity when applied to the skin; this has led to severely restricted use and a complete ban is possible, although many oppose this view.
- The identified allergens include atranorin, chloroatronin and haematomates.

Compare with

- Tree moss absolute: complex, warm, earthy, mossy, phenolic, woody and herbaceous. Tree moss lichens include *Evernia furfuraceae* and *Usnea barbata*, which grow on conifers – spruce, fir and pine – so the piney, coniferous, resinous odours of these trees can be detected in the lichen and tree moss absolute.

Agrestic Family

Patchouli essential oil

Botanical source

Pogostemon cablin semi-dried and lightly fermented leaves

Odour profile

TYPE: patchouli

CHARACTERISTICS: rich, intense, rounded, smooth, persistent, slightly sweet

SUBSIDIARY NOTES AND NUANCES: earthy, balsamic, woody, spicy, rooty, herbaceous, green, bitter chocolate, peppery, wine-like

Olfactory notes

- The oil has a very distinctive odour, aromatic and with considerable persistence. Look for the contrasts: light and shade; the fresh and slightly herbal top notes, compared with the richness in the body; its almost sweet nature compared with slight bitterness which is harmonised by the balsamic and almost chocolate-like nuances.

- It is unusual in that it improves with age.

- The chemistry of patchouli oil is very complex; however, the dominant constituents are the sesquiterpene alcohols, especially patchoulol (very weak odour) and norpatchoulenol (patchouli-like), and sesquiterpenes including α- and β-bulnesene, patchoulene, α-guaiene and caryophyllene (woody, spicy, clove-like).

- Patchouli oil is extremely important in the fragrance industry.

- The oil is also used as a food flavour in sweets, baked goods and even some meats and sausages.

- The tar content of tobacco and cigarettes has been reduced by many manufacturers, and this has affected the flavour of the products, so patchouli oil is sometimes added to compensate for the changed flavour.

Compare with

- Vetiver essential oil: preferably from Réunion; has a smooth, strong, sweet, rich, woody and earthy aroma, with rooty, musty nuances reminiscent of sliced raw potato. From *Vetiveria zizanoides* rootlets; patchouli shares several of its sensory qualities.

- Hay absolute: also rich, warm and sweet with hay and green notes. From *Hierochloe alpina* dried grass.

- Cacao absolute: this has a rich, warm, balsamic scent that is reminiscent of chocolate, but minus the vanilla; obtained from *Theobroma cacao*.

Tobacco leaf absolute

Botanical source

Nicotiana tabacum semi-dried leaves

Odour profile

TYPE: tabac

CHARACTERISTICS: rich, intense, warm, slightly sweet

SUBSIDIARY NOTES AND NUANCES: hay, green

Olfactory notes

- Tobacco concrete, absolute and resinoid are also used in the fragrance industry to obtain genuine tabac notes.
- The tabac note has been described as being like that of cured pipe tobacco.
- Undiluted, the absolute can be perceived as strong and unpleasant; it is only described as 'mellow' if in dilution.
- Constituents include the phenolic compounds *para*-cresol (tar-like, narcissus-like), *para*-ethyl phenol, guaiacols (phenolic, smoky), eugenol (clove-like), tobacco acids and esters; may contain traces of nicotine.

Compare with

- Hay absolute: also rich, warm and sweet with hay and green notes; from *Hierochloe alpina* dried grass.
- Tonka bean absolute: rich, sweet, warm, subtle, hay-like with herbaceous, vanillic and coconut-like nuances; used as a fixative. The botanical source is *Dipteryx odorata* beans. Tobacco absolute demonstrates a different kind of sweetness – it is not vanilla-like, but it is very compatible with this type of aroma.
- Coffee absolute: has an aroma very similar to roasted coffee beans – deep, rich, warm and earthy; from *Coffea arabica* roasted beans. Tobacco leaf absolute shares the deep, rich, warm characteristics, but is hay-like and green as opposed to earthy.
- Cacao absolute: this has a rich, warm, balsamic scent that is reminiscent of chocolate, but minus the vanilla; obtained from *Theobroma cacao*. Compare the rich, warm cacao characteristics with coffee absolute too.

Agrestic Family

22

Floral Family

Champaca absolute

Botanical source

Michaelia champaca (golden yellow) or *M. alba* (white) flowers

Odour profile

TYPE: floral

CHARACTERISTICS: penetrating, sweet, heady, warm, smooth and rich

SUBSIDIARY NOTES AND NUANCES: neroli, orange flower, lily, hay, fruity, spicy, tea-like

Olfactory notes

- Champaca is often used in jasmine fragrances.
- The absolute is very scarce.
- Over 250 constituents have been reported, including linalool (sweet, fresh floral and woody), methyl benzoate (sweet, fruity, heavy floral, ylang ylang), benzyl acetate (fruity, jasmine-like), phenylethanol (honey, rosy), α-ionone and β-ionone (violet-like), methyl anthranilate (orange-flower-like, fruity, harsh) and indole (animalic).
- Indole is a cyclic imine: a nitrogen-containing molecule – and is a trace constituent in the volatile oil of some white flowers; it is very important in their aroma. It has been described as faecal at 10 per cent and it can be perceived as the odour of putrefaction, but trace amounts can impart a jasmine-like effect.

Compare with

- Jasmine absolute: intense, diffusive, heavy, warm and rich, floral, with fruity, green, tea-like and indolic nuances; from *Jasminum grandiflorum* flowers.
- Orange blossom absolute: fresh top, heady, intense, rich and heavy orange flower, with indolic, animalic and green nuances; from *Citrus aurantium* var. *amara* flowers.
- Ylang ylang extra essential oil: sweet, heady, persistent, diffusive and floral, with a fruity character, medicated and creamy nuances; lacks the indolic facet. The botanical source is *Cananga odorata* var. *genuina* flowers.

Frangipani absolute

Botanical source

Plumeria species, including *P. rubra* (red) and *P. acuminata* (white) flowers

Odour profile

TYPE: floral (tropical)

CHARACTERISTICS: diffusive, strong, heady, sweet, rich

SUBSIDIARY NOTES AND NUANCES: honey, fruity, spicy, green, citrus

Olfactory notes

- The strongly scented *Plumeria* varieties can be described in terms of other fragrance types such as citrus, coconut, rose, cinnamon, carnation, jasmine, gardenia, fruity and woody.

- The composition is complex and variable; however, the absolutes are rich in esters, notably benzyl salicylate (mild, sweet, floral-balsamic), neryl phenylacetate (fruity, rosy and apple-like), benzyl salicylate (faint, sweet, floral), phenyl ethyl benzoate (faint, floral, balsamic) and phenyl ethyl cinnamate (rosy, honey-like); also *trans*-nerolidol (mild, pleasant floral odour), linalool (mild, woody, floral) and geranial (citrus notes).

Compare with

- Aglaia absolute: light and fresh floral, with jasmine and lemon-like notes; from *Aglaia odorata* flowers.
- Jasmine absolute: intense, diffusive, heavy, warm and rich, floral, with fruity, green, tea-like and indolic nuances; from *Jasminum grandiflorum* flowers.
- Rose absolute: rich, sweet, smooth floral (rose) with honey and spicy nuances; from *Rosa centifolia* flowers.
- Osmanthus absolute: rich, sweet, honey-like and fruity, with plum, raisin and apricot nuances; from *Osmanthus fragrans* flowers.

Floral Family

Genet absolute

Botanical source

Spartium junceum flowers

Odour profile

TYPE: floral (green)

CHARACTERISTICS: persistent, sweet, warm, slightly harsh if undiluted

SUBSIDIARY NOTES AND NUANCES: rosy, green, herbaceous, hay

Olfactory notes

- Genet absolute is obtained from the Spanish broom.
- The fresh flowers have a sweet scent reminiscent of orange blossom and musty grapes.
- An absolute is also obtained from the common broom, *Cytisus scoparius.*
- Genet absolute is complex and contains esters such as ethyl myristate (mild, violet-like), ethyl palmitate (light, waxy, sweet), ethyl oleate (weak floral), and linalyl acetate (fresh, sweet, fruity); and alcohols such as linalool (mild floral, woody), phenyl ethanol (sweet, honey-like, rosy).
- Broom has been used as a perfume ingredient since the 16th century.

Compare with

- Broom absolute: sweet, green, floral and honey-like; from the common broom, *Cytisus scoparius.*
- Mimosa absolute: soft, sweet, delicate green floral; from *Acacia dealbata* flowers.
- Narcissus absolute: heavy, sweet, herbaceous, hay-like, earthy, floral odour; it only smells like narcissus on extreme dilution. The botanical source is *Narcissus poeticus.*

Jasmine absolute

Botanical sources

Jasminum grandiflorum and *J. sambac* flowers

Odour profile

J. grandiflorum from France:

> TYPE: floral (jasmine), indolic
>
> CHARACTERISTICS: heady, intense, diffusive, rich and heavy, warm
>
> SUBSIDIARY NOTES AND NUANCES: fruity, animalic, waxy, spicy, tea-like, green

J. sambac from India:

> TYPE: floral (jasmine)
>
> CHARACTERISTICS: sweet, delicate, fresh, light top notes, but body is heady, intense, diffusive, rich
>
> SUBSIDIARY NOTES AND NUANCES: lily-like, tea-like, fruity, green

Olfactory notes

- Dominated by aromatic esters such as benzyl acetate (fresh, jasmine-like, fruity), methyl jasmonate (sweet, floral, herbaceous), methyl anthranilate (orange-flower-like, fruity, harsh) and benzyl benzoate (faint, sweet, balsamic); monoterpenoid alcohols such as linalool (sweet, fresh floral, woody) are present, as are aromatic alcohols such as benzyl alcohol (almost odourless) and the sesquiterpenol farnesol (delicate floral, lily-of-the-valley-like); the celery-like ketone *cis*-jasmone is also found, and trace amounts of indole.

- Indole is a cyclic imine (a nitrogen-containing molecule) and a trace constituent in the volatile oil of some white flowers; it is very important in their aroma. Described as faecal at 10 per cent, it can be perceived as the odour of putrefaction, but trace amounts can impart a jasmine-like effect.

Compare with

- Orange blossom absolute: fresh top, heady, intense, rich and heavy orange flower, with animalic and green nuances; from *Citrus aurantium* var. *amara* flowers.

- White champaca absolute: penetrating, heady, warm, smooth and rich, with a similarity to lily; orange flower/neroli-like and spicy, hay and tea-like undertones. From *Michelia alba* flowers.

- Ylang ylang extra essential oil: sweet, heady, persistent, diffusive and floral, with a fruity character, medicated and creamy nuances. The botanical source is *Cananga odorata* var. *genuina* flowers.

Linden blossom absolute

Botanical source

Tilea vulgaris flowers

Odour profile

TYPE: floral (green type)

CHARACTERISTICS: fresh, delicate

SUBSIDARY NOTES AND NUANCES: honey, broom, white lilac, lily of the valley, lily, hay

Olfactory notes

- Dominated by farnesol (also found in lesser amounts in mimosa and cassie absolutes, and many other floral absolutes); this contributes the sweet, delicate, floral, linden-blossom-like, lily-of-the-valley-like notes.

- A CO_2 extract has become available; this is said to be closer to the powerful scent of fresh linden flowers.

Compare with

- Mimosa absolute: soft, sweet, delicate, green, floral; from *Acacia dealbata* flowers. Also contains farnesol.

- Genet absolute: tenacious, sweet, floral (rosy), with green, herbaceous and hay notes; from the flowers of *Spartium junceum*.

Mimosa absolute

Botanical source

Acacia dealbata flowers and twig ends

Odour profile

TYPE: floral (green type)

CHARACTERISTICS: soft, sweet, rich, delicate

SUBSIDARY NOTES AND NUANCES: woody, waxy, honey, hawthorn blossom

Olfactory notes

- In Grasse in France *La Fête du Mimosa* is held every February to celebrate the delicately scented golden flowers that represent the end of winter.

- Mimosa flowers have a delicate scent, candyfloss- and honey-like, but balanced with a sharper green note.

- One of its main constituents is farnesol, a sesquiterpene alcohol with a sweet, delicate, floral, linden-blossom-like, lily-of-the-valley-like odour.

- It also contains phenylethanol (sweet, honey, rose), aldehydes C_9 (floral, waxy fruity) and C_{10} (sweet, fruity, citrus), *cis*-3-hexenyl acetate (fresh, green, fruity, banana-like), benzaldehyde (sweet, powerful, bitter-almond-like), ethyl benzoate (warm, smooth, fruity-floral), linalool (mild, woody, floral), anethole (sweet, warm, herbaceous, like star anise), *cis*-jasmone (fruity and celery-seed-like, on dilution reminiscent of jasmine), anisaldehyde (powerful, sweet, reminiscent of hawthorn blossom) and 2-*trans*-6-*cis*-nonadien-1-al (diffusive, leafy green, cucumber-like).

- In perfumery mimosa is often used in lilac, lily of the valley and violet type fragrances.

Compare with

- Cassie absolute: warm, floral, with a delicate, powdery, violet-like top and herbaceous, spicy nuances and balsamic base notes. (The balsamic note is not present in mimosa.) From *Acacia farnesiana* flowers. Cassie also contains farnesol.

- Linden blossom absolute: delicate, green, floral, with honey nuances; dominated by farnesol. From *Tilea vulgaris* flowers.

Floral Family

Narcissus absolute

Botanical source

Narcissus poeticus flowers

Odour profile

TYPE: floral

CHARACTERISTICS: heavy, sweet, narcotic

SUBSIDIARY NOTES AND NUANCES: earthy, herbaceous, hay-like

Olfactory notes

- The genus *Narcissus* contains *N. pseudo-narcissus* (daffodil), *N. jonquilla* (jonquil) and *N. poeticus* (narcissus), from which an essential oil (by enfleurage) and an absolute can be obtained.
- An absolute is also obtained from jonquil.
- Narcissus absolute is used in perfumery; it has a tiny yield, but is produced in small quantities mainly in the Lozère, in the Languedoc Roussillon region of France.
- It only smells like narcissus on extreme dilution.
- A complex composition, containing phenylethanol (sweet, honey, rosy), α-terpineol (lilac-like), *l*-linalool (mild floral, woody), γ-methyl ionone (soft, rich, violet-like, woody, leafy), anisaldehyde (sweet, hawthorn blossom, hay) and benzyl acetate (fresh, fruity, floral, jasmine-like) and trace amounts of indole.

Compare with

- Broom absolute: sweet, green floral and honey-like; from the common broom, *Cytisus scoparius*.
- Mimosa absolute: soft, sweet, delicate green floral; from *Acacia dealbata* flowers.
- Jonquil absolute: fresh top, heavy, narcotic, sweet, honey, green floral odour; similar to narcissus. The botanical source is the rush daffodil, *Narcissus jonquilla*.
- Hyacinth absolute: a very powerful, sharp, green, leaf-like odour, pleasant only on dilution, and only resembling hyacinth on extreme dilution; narcotic qualities. From *Hyacinthus orientalis* flowers. The absolute is scarce; synthetic hyacinth lacks the deep green/earthy note, and sweet, green floral notes dominate.

Orange blossom absolute

Botanical source

Citrus aurantium var. *amara* flowers

Odour profile

TYPE: floral (orange flower), indolic

CHARACTERISTICS: fresh top, heady, intense, rich and heavy body and dryout

SUBSIDIARY NOTES AND NUANCES: green, animalic, faecal

Olfactory notes

- Orange blossom absolute is very important in perfumery, contributing to the heart of fragrances (often the 'white flowers' type).

- Only when diluted does the absolute smell like the flowers.

- It is dominated by linalool (fresh floral and woody), linalyl acetate (fresh, light, herbal and fruity/pear drops), nerolidol (delicate, floral, green), farnesol (delicate, sweet, floral and green), and also contains the rosy-scented phenylethanol and methyl anthranilate (orange flower, fruity, dry), which is a nitrogen-containing ester also found in mandarin oil.

- Orange blossom absolute contains traces of indole; in its pure form this smells like mothballs, a naphthalene-like odour, and at 10 per cent concentration it has been described as faecal; this constituent is thought to contribute to the animalic/faecal nuance.

- Indole is a cyclic imine – a nitrogen-containing molecule – and is a trace constituent in the volatile oil of some white flowers; it is very important in their aroma. It can be perceived as the odour of putrefaction, but trace amounts can impart a jasmine-like effect.

Compare with

- Neroli bigarade essential oil: light, orange-flower floral, with slightly bitter herbaceous and green notes; the distilled counterpart of orange blossom absolute.

- Tuberose absolute: a heavy, sweet, honey-like, sweet-caramel, indolic floral. See if you can detect green notes and nuances of camphor, rubber and even rotting meat (indole). From *Polyanthus tuberosa* flowers.

- Jasmine absolute: intense, diffusive, heavy, warm and rich, floral, with fruity, green, tea-like and indolic nuances. From *Jasminum grandiflorum* flowers.

Floral Family

Osmanthus absolute

Botanical source

Osmanthus fragrans flowers

Odour profile

TYPE: floral (fruity)

CHARACTERISTICS: sweet, rich, complex

SUBSIDIARY NOTES AND NUANCES: honey, dried fruit, raisins, plums, apricots

Olfactory notes

- Sweet osmanthus, also known as *kweiha*, is one of the ten traditional flowers of China.
- The flowers can vary in colour according to type, from silvery-white to reddish-orange; golden-orange-yellow flowers are regarded as having the best scent.
- Osmanthus has an interesting and complex floral-fruity dynamic.
- Constituents that are important in its odour are β-ionone (woody, floral, violet, slightly fruity, with cedarwood, raspberry nuances); dihydro-β-ionone, γ-decalactone (powerful, peach-like) and related lactones; linalool (light floral, woody), nerol (sweet, floral, seaweed-like) and geraniol (sweet, rosy)

Compare with

- Frangipani (*Plumeria rubra* varieties) absolute: sweet and tea-rose-like, with spicy-herbaceous notes. Methyl salicylate is present in some varieties and may (along with other constituents) contribute to the sweet, spicy/herbaceous/fruity nuances.
- Red champaca absolute: sweet, complex, fruity floral (jasmine-like), again showing a floral-fruity dynamic, but with emphasis on the floral aspect; from the flowers of red *Michelia champaca* varieties.

Pink lotus absolute

Botanical source

Nelumbo nucifera flowers

Odour profile

TYPE: floral

CHARACTERISTICS: rich, sweet, aromatic

SUBSIDIARY NOTES AND NUANCES: fruity, herbaceous, leathery, powdery, spicy, muddy, medicated

Olfactory notes

- The lotus is an aquatic perennial, with scented blue, white or white and pink-tipped flowers.
- There are several cultivars, but they all have similar scents.
- The absolute is complex and constituents include caryophyllene oxide, β-caryophyllene (light, spicy, clove-like, woody) and *cis*-jasmone (fruity and celery-seed-like; on dilution it is reminiscent of jasmine).
- A medicated note has been observed; this is contributed by 1,4-dimethoxybenzene.
- Lotus absolute needs to mature in order to develop its fragrance.
- *Nelumbo lutea* is the yellow-flowering American lotus, and it has a more pronounced jasmine note.
- White lotus is a dark brown, viscous liquid with a similar odour but an animalic, herbaceous dryout.

Compare with

- White lotus absolute: rich, sweet, aromatic and floral, but with an animalic and herbaceous dryout.

Rose absolute

Botanical source

Rosa centifolia (France) and *R. damascena* (Bulgaria) flowers

Odour profile

TYPE: rose

CHARACTERISTICS: rich, sweet, smooth

SUBSIDIARY NOTES AND NUANCES: waxy, honey, spicy

Olfactory notes

- Rose is extremely important in perfumery, and often used with synthetic rose aromachemicals to give a natural effect.
- The absolute contributes to the middle (heart) notes of a fragrance.
- French (and Moroccan) rose absolute from *R. centifolia* is often called 'Rose de Mai'.
- Rose absolute is dominated by the rose alcohols – phenylethyl alcohol (soft, petal-like, rosy), citronellol (warm and vibrant rosy), geraniol (sharper rosy) and nerol (harsher and fresh rosy), which occur in varying proportions depending on species and variety; it also contains farnesol, which contributes sweet, delicate, floral and green nuances.
- An essential oil (otto) is also produced, usually from *R. damascena*. The otto contributes to the top rather than the middle notes of a fragrance; characterised by geraniol and citronellol, and only small amounts of phenylethanol.

Compare with

- Rose otto: deep, sweet, warm, rich, rosy, waxy; less spicy than the absolute, and the Moroccan oil is in turn less spicy than oils from Bulgaria or Turkey.
- Geranium (Bourbon) essential oil: fresh, rosy with herbaceous, green, vegetable and minty nuances; from the leaves of *Pelargonium graveolens* (also *P. capitatum* × *P. radens* (rose geranium) and *P. capitatum* × *P. graveolens* hybrids).
- Immortelle absolute: sweet, herbaceous, floral (rosy), with spicy, hay, honey and woody nuances; from *Helichrysum angustifolium* flowers.
- Palmarosa essential oil: fresh, sweet, delicate, floral (rosy), with woody, violet and oily nuances; from the grass-like leaves of *Cymbopogon martinii* var. *martinii*.
- Guaiacwood essential oil: soft, sweet, clean, tea rose, woody and balsamic; from *Bulnesia sarmientoi* wood.

Ylang ylang extra essential oil

Botanical source

Cananga odorata var. *genuina* flowers

Odour profile

TYPE: floral (tropical)

CHARACTERISTICS: diffusive, strong, sweet, heady, smooth and rich

SUBSIDIARY NOTES AND NUANCES: fruity, medicated, spicy

Olfactory notes

- The term 'extra' indicates that the oil is from the first fraction of the distillation, and is considered to have the finest odour; 'No. 3', the last fraction of the distillation process, is also used in perfumery.
- The 'complete' distillate is sold as cananga oil.
- 'Extra' is complex, and contains linalool (sweet, fresh floral and woody), methyl acetate (sweet, floral, minty), methyl benzoate (sweet, fruity, heavy floral, ylang ylang), benzyl acetate (fruity, jasmine-like), benzyl salicylate (sweet, floral, balsamic), geranyl acetate (sweet, rose- and lavender-like), and methyl salicylate (fruity, medicated), *para*-cresyl methyl ether (pungent and ylang-ylang-like), caryophyllene (spicy, clove-like and woody) and *iso*-eugenol (warm, tenacious, carnation- and wallflower-like). It has higher levels of *para*-cresyl methyl ether (in dilution similar to narcissus and ylang-ylang), methyl benzoate (heavy floral, ylang-ylang-like), linalool, methyl acetate and geranyl acetate than the other grades.
- Has potential for skin sensitisation.

Compare with

- Cananga essential oil: sweet, floral, with medicated, woody and oily nuances; from *Cananga odorata* flowers.
- Ylang ylang absolute: very similar odour profile to the essential oil, but rounder and softer.
- Jasmine absolute: intense, diffusive, heavy, warm and rich, floral, with fruity, green, tea-like and indolic nuances; from *Jasminum grandiflorum* flowers.
- Frangipani absolute: rich, exotic, heady floral aroma, with sweet, honey-like notes and fruity notes; from *Plumeria* species.

23

Fruity Family

Blackcurrant bud absolute

Botanical source

Ribes nigrum flower buds

Odour profile

TYPE: fruity, green

CHARACTERISTICS: strong, diffusive, penetrating

SUBSIDIARY NOTES AND NUANCES: herbal, blackcurrant, minty, catty

Olfactory notes

- Blackcurrant bud is difficult to categorise; it has a unique odour profile mainly because of the catty nuance, and also because of the balance between fruity and green.
- In the perfumery industry blackcurrant bud is known as *bourgeons de cassissier*, or *cassis bourgeons*.
- In perfumery the fruity green notes in blackcurrant bud can be used to modify intense green odours, such as that of galbanum and violet leaf.
- The 'catty' element is, for some, reminiscent of male cat's urine or the sexually related odour of the male cat.
- The catty element is partly contributed by trace amounts of sulphur compounds, specifically a thiole named 4-methoxy-2-methylbutan-2-thiol, which is reputed to have an olfactory detection threshold of 1 in 1,000,000 billion.

Compare with

- Tagetes essential oil: pungent, warm, sweet, fruity (apple-like) and herbaceous, with minty nuances; from *Tagetes glandulifera* aerial parts.

Roman chamomile essential oil

Botanical source

Anthemis nobilis flowers

Odour profile

TYPE: fruity (herbal)

CHARACTERISTICS: sweet, warm, intense, diffusive

SUBSIDIARY NOTES AND NUANCES: herbaceous, apple-like, tea-like

Olfactory notes

- Dominated by non-terpenoid esters such as *iso*-butyl angelate and related esters (herbal and fruity), and esters of tiglic acid (herbal and fruity).

- It is occasionally used in perfumery, but in small amounts and mainly in chypre type fragrances.

- With regard to the relationship between green notes and fruity notes, it has been suggested that trace amounts of the lower fruity esters, such as those in Roman chamomile, can modify the harshness of some green materials like galbanum and violet leaf.

Compare with

- Roman chamomile absolute: sweet, warm, fruity and herbal, but more robust, sweeter and warmer, and also slightly floral.

- German chamomile essential oil: sweet, herbal and fruity, with hay notes and a tobacco-like nuance in the drydown; from *Chamomilla recutita* dried flowers.

- Tagetes essential oil: pungent, warm, sweet, fruity (apple-like) and herbaceous with minty nuances; from *Tagetes glandulifera* aerial parts.

Tagetes essential oil

Botanical source

Tagetes minuta flowering tops

Odour profile

TYPE: fruity (apple)

CHARACTERISTICS: warm, sweet, pungent, can be harsh

SUBSIDIARY NOTES AND NUANCES: green, apple (especially when diluted), herbaceous, minty

Olfactory notes

- The fresh oil is a liquid; however, it thickens and becomes sticky with age and exposure to the air.

- The main constituents are ketones: *cis*-tagetone, *trans*-tagetone and dihydrotagetone (which impart warm and herbal notes); also *l*-linalool (mild, floral, woody) and ocimene (light, warm and herbaceous). It contains traces of non-volatile furanocoumarins (psoralen) and perhaps other compounds which cause phototoxicity; the levels of tagetes oil are restricted in perfumery.

Compare with

- Roman chamomile essential oil: sweet, warm, fruity (apple-like) and herbaceous; from *Anthemis nobilis* flowers.

- Blackcurrant bud absolute: strong, green and fruity (blackcurrant) with herbaceous and catty notes; from *Ribes nigrum* flower buds.

24

Citrus (Hesperidic) Family

Bergamot essential oil

Botanical source

Citrus aurantium subsp. *bergamia* fruit peel

Odour profile

TYPE: citrus

CHARACTERISTICS: sharp top, sweet, rich

SUBSIDIARY NOTES AND NUANCES: lemon, floral, peppery, herbaceous

Olfactory notes

- The most important citrus oil from the fragrance perspective.
- Does not have the typical citrus, zesty aroma of the other citrus peel oils, but has a floral (freesia-like) quality, which some say is reminiscent of lavender and neroli.
- There is a great deal of variation in its composition, usually related to its geographical origins.
- The major components are alcohols such as *l*-linalool (mild, floral, woody), esters including linalyl acetate (floral and fruity), and monoterpenes including *d*-limonene (fresh, weak citrus), α- and β-pinene (resinous, fresh and pine-like) and γ-terpinene (terpeney, sweet, citrus scent with tropical and lime nuances).
- Bergamot is an essential component of eau de cologne type fragrances, usually with lemon, orange, petitgrain, neroli, and often rosemary and rose.
- Bergamot is extremely versatile, and appears in all of the other fragrance categories.
- Along with oakmoss and labdanum, bergamot is important in the chypre structure and so it is found in most chypres, especially the fresh type.

Compare with

- Yuzu essential oil: strong, aromatic citrus with floral nuances; from *C. × junos*, a hybrid of *C. ichangensis* (the Ichang lemon or papeda) and the sour mandarin.
- Petitgrain essential oil: petitgrain 'bigarade' has a fresh, floral, sweet, orange-citrus scent with bitter herbal and woody nuances; from *C. aurantium* subsp. *amara* leaves and twigs.
- Lavender essential oil: sweet, fresh, light herbal, with soft floral, fruity and woody nuances; from *Lavandula angustifolia* flowering tops.
- Neroli bigarade essential oil: light orange flower floral, with slightly bitter herbaceous and green notes; from *C. aurantium* subsp. *amara* flowers.

Cédrat essential oil

Botanical source

Citrus medica peel

Odour profile

TYPE: citrus

CHARACTERISTICS: sharp, intense, deep, relatively tenacious

SUBSIDIARY NOTES AND NUANCES: green, lemon

Olfactory notes

- *Citrus medica* is one of the ancestral citrus species; others such as the lemon are descended from it.
- It resembles a large lemon, but the pulp is dry and there is a considerable amount of pith that adheres to the segments.
- Known as the citron, or the French cédrat of perfumery; valued for its tenacity and depth in comparison to most other citrus oils.
- As with most citrus oils, the immediate impact is given by *d*-limonene, which evaporates first, giving a fresh, sharp, citrus impression; then the moderately volatile components, present in smaller amounts, such as the aldehyde citral (lemony), and esters such as geranyl acetate (sweet, rosy, fruity) start to evaporate, their odours mingling with that of *d*-limonene and the other terpenes such as β-pinene (fresh, pine), and γ-terpinene (terpeney, sweet, citrus); the aroma therefore becomes stronger and more pronounced, sweeter and fruitier, and less sharp.
- Cold-pressed citrus oils often contain furanocoumarins, which are constituents that are implicated in phototoxicity.

Compare with

- Bitter orange cold-pressed essential oil: fresh and delicate citrus, with sweet floral and green notes; more subtle and fresh than sweet orange, with a greater degree of tenacity than most other citrus oils (comparable with cédrat); from the peel of *C. aurantium* var. *amara*.
- Grapefruit cold-pressed essential oil: sharp citrus top notes, sweet, fresh citrus, orange-like body, but distinctively grapefruit due to traces of a sulphur-containing compound called nootkatone; from the peel of *C. paradisi.*
- Lime distilled essential oil: fresh, sharp, terpenic top with a sweet, fruity, citrus, typically lime, character; from the peel of *C. aurantifolia.*
- Lemon cold-pressed essential oil: fresh, sharp citrus top with a sweet, fresh lemony body; from *C. limonum*, or *C. limon* peel.

Mandarin essential oil

Botanical source

Citrus reticulata peel

Odour profile

TYPE: citrus

CHARACTERISTICS: intense, sweet, soft

SUBSIDIARY NOTES AND NUANCES: fruity, orange-like, occasionally amine (fishy)

Olfactory notes

- Mandarin and tangerine are usually considered as one species; however, the mandarin, *C. reticulata*, originated in China, and the tangerine may be a hybrid species, *C. × tangerina*.
- 'Tangerine' is the name used in English-speaking countries, and 'mandarin' elsewhere.
- The unripe, green fruits yield the oil that is preferred in perfumery; this is light yellow in colour. When the fruits reach the final stage of maturity the oil will be red or orange in colour, depending on how it has been extracted; mandarin is therefore sold as green, yellow or red. The chemical composition of the oil will vary too.
- An amine (fishy) note can be present due to the presence of nitrogen-containing compounds such as trimethylamine.
- Dominated by *d*-limonene (fresh, weak citrus), other terpenes including γ-terpinene (terpeney, sweet, citrus scent with tropical and lime nuances), α- and β-pinene (fresh, resinous, pine-like), myrcene (sweet and balsamic); also alcohols, short chain fatty aldehydes C_8 (sharp, fatty, fruity, sweet orange-like), C_{10} (citrus fruity, sweet orange-like), C_{12} (waxy, floral, violet, sweet, fresh), trace amounts of thymol (medicated, herbaceous) and methyl-*N*-methyl anthranilate (orange flower, heavy, fruity, mandarin-like).

Compare with

- Sweet orange cold-pressed essential oil: light, fresh, citrus, fruity top notes, and the middle is citrus, fruity and aldehydic; from the peel of *C. sinensis, C. aurantium* var. *dulce*.
- *C. tachibana* cold-pressed essential oil: sweet, green citrus; related to mandarin.

Litsea cubeba essential oil

Botanical source

Litsea cubeba small fruits

Odour profile

TYPE: lemon

CHARACTERISTICS: fresh, sweet, intense, sharp

SUBSIDIARY NOTES AND NUANCES: fruity

Olfactory notes

- Also called may chang and tropical verbena; lemon notes contributed by citral (strong lemon), *d*-limonene (weak citrus), *d*-citronellal (powerful fresh, green lemon odour faint with rosy herbaceous undertones) and methyl heptenone (green, fruity, oily, harsh).
- Citral is the name given to the naturally occurring isomers neral and geranial. The citral found in citrus oils has a slightly different odour from citral found in other lemon-scented botanicals, including *Litsea cubeba* because of the relative proportions of the isomers.
- The oil is used for the isolation of citral and the synthesis of violet-scented ionones from this. In industrial perfumery it is used to impart lemon odour to middle notes.

Compare with

- Citronella essential oil: sweet, fresh, lemony, from *Cymbopogon winterianus* (Java); or lemony, floral, grassy and woody (Ceylon); dominated by citronellal.
- Combava petityrain (kaffir lime leaf): citronellar-like, lime and floral-rosy notes; from the leaves of *Citrus hystrix*.
- Lemon-scented eucalyptus essential oil: strong, fresh, rosy-citronella; from *Eucalyptus citriodora* leaves and twiglets; dominated by citronellal.
- Lemon-scented ironbark essential oil: sweet, fresh, fruity-lemon, verbena-like scent; from *Eucalyptus staigeriana* leaves and twiglets; the lemony odour is due to neral.
- Lemongrass essential oil: tenacious, strong, lemony, herbal aroma, with a herbal, oily dryout; from *Cymbopogon citratus* or *C. flexuosus* grass.
- Lemon-scented tea tree essential oil: distinctive lemony, pungent, diffusive odour; from leaves and twigs of *Leptospermum petersonii*; contains both citral and citronellal.
- Melissa essential oil: citrus, herbal top notes, and a herbal body; from the leaves of *Melissa officinalis*; dominated by citral.

Citrus (Hesperidic) Family

Part III

AN EXPERIENTIAL PROGRAMME OF STUDY

25

Reset Your Nose with Scents in the Natural World

Take in the forest atmosphere – shinrin-yoku

Shinrin-yoku translates as 'forest bathing', or 'taking in the forest atmosphere', and the practice has been shown to have remarkable health benefits. Tsunetsugu, Park and Miyazaki (2010) have investigated the physiological effects of exposure to the 'total environment' of forests, including deciduous broad-leafed forests as well as conifer-dominated ones, and also the physiological effects of certain elements (such as the odour of the forest, some essential oils derived from forest species, the sound of running streams, and the scenery). Their work has confirmed that *shinrin-yoku* can reduce stress, reduce blood glucose levels in diabetic patients, increase natural killer cell activity and immunoglobulins A, G and M, reduce feelings of hostility and depression, and lower blood pressure. They suggest that *shinrin-yoku* is 'forest medicine' and that the practice could make a significant contribution to human health (see Colour Plates 3 and 4).

So next time you take a walk in the woods, be aware of how you are feeling and the enormous benefits it can bring. Seek out the coniferous aroma in conifer forests and pine woods, and how this compares with, for example, an oak wood or a birch community. Look for the smell of geosmin, which gives the aroma of damp earth and the smell in the air after rain has fallen. In spring, some trees such as the linden produce delicately scented flowers, so take the opportunity to smell these if you can. In the late spring, you might find the very beautiful lily of the valley (*Convallaria majalis*) growing wild in the forests and wooded glades of Europe. Its tiny, bell-shaped, white flowers have a delicate, green, rosy-floral scent. In the autumn, can you detect the smell of fungi, decaying wood and leaves?

Walk along the sea shore

The sea shore can deliver some unique sensations, depending on the landscape, weather, tides and waters (see Colour Plates 5 and 6). It is really very difficult to describe the smell of the sea, let alone define what constitutes it. For many years there was a popular notion that we smelt ozone – a molecule comprised of three oxygen atoms – which was responsible for the clean and bracing air at the seaside. It is not healthy to inhale ozone in high concentrations, and it has a faint chlorine-like smell that we can detect it in the air after a thunderstorm or heavy rainfall; some liken it to the smell around a photocopier. However, we now know that ozone has very little to do with the smell of sea air; instead we need to consider what is in the natural environment that contributes to the smell, or sensation. It could be sand, salt, sea creatures, algae, plankton, ocean bacteria and seaweed, and their metabolites, in a myriad combinations. One of the main contenders is actually a gas – dimethyl sulphide, or DMS. This is produced by ocean-dwelling bacteria that colonise dying plankton and seaweeds, and in the natural environment it has a fishy, tangy smell. DMS attracts seabirds – it may be a homing scent, or an aid to finding food. It is also involved in cloud formation, and therefore has a very important role in the ecosystem. We have a low olfactory threshold for DMS, which is often described as cabbage-like, and indeed it is released by several vegetables when they are cooked, before being oxidised in the atmosphere. It is also found in black truffles.

Seaweed will have a large part to play in the smell on the beach of a sea loch. *Laminaria digitata* is very common in the British Isles and abundant on the west coast of Scotland. It is large, with olive-coloured leathery fronds, attaching to rocks that lie below the ordinary tides. It has a strong characteristic smell, more noticeable when the tide is out, or when it is washed up on the shore and begins to decay.

The sand dunes that border some beaches are host to the fragrant common broom, which has a sweet and honey-like aroma, and in Scotland gorse grows well in coastal areas; when it is in bloom the air is filled with its pineapple-like scent!

Stroll through meadows and hedgerows

Pastures, meadows and hedgerows offer a special olfactory opportunity! You might detect a sweet, honey-like scent from sweet alyssum (*Alyssum compactum*) and sweet-scented vernal grass (*Anthoxanthum odoratum*), which is widespread in pastures and hayfields in the southeast of the USA. Also known as vanilla grass, holy grass and buffalo grass, it too has a sweet smell reminiscent of hay and vanilla. The alpine sweetgrass (*Hierochloe alpina*) is also very beautiful.

Sweet clover (*Melilotus officinalis*) is a fragrant perennial herb that is very attractive to bees, which also flourishes in meadows and pastures. As its name suggests, this too has a sweet scent that is reminiscent of new-mown hay, but also of woodruff. When in flower, the heady, sweet and honey-like perfume of meadowsweet (*Filipendula ulmaria*) is part of the scent of the meadows; the plant is found growing along streams and in the hedgerows which border fields and pastures. You can also look for hawthorn blossom. Hawthorn (*Cratageus oxycantha*) is a very common hedge tree in Europe. Its small flowers have snowy white petals and bright pink stamens, and they have a heady, intoxicating, sweet, rich scent. These aromatic species all contribute to a happy and uplifting atmosphere, and so it is not surprising that many of us like to spend time in the places where they grow. Hay fever sufferers are, unfortunately, at a disadvantage!

Spend some quality olfactory time with flowers in the garden

This, of course, depends on where in the world you live, or can visit (see Colour Plates 7 and 8)! In Europe we can enjoy the way honeysuckle (*Lonicera periclymenum* and *L. caprifolium*) flowers fill the air with scent on a summer evening; or bathe in the sweet, all-encompassing fragrance of night-scented stocks, or the sweet, diffusive perfume of the tiny flowers of *Eleagnus*; or experience the heady lilac and the soft, clove-like carnation (*Dianthus caryophyllus* and *D. plumarius*), the sumptuous peony (there are several scented *Paeonia* species), the lily (try *Lilium candidum* and some of the 'Turk's cap' types); and, of course, the rose with its many glorious aromas! If you can, look for a scented hybrid tea rose (such as 'Fragrant Cloud'), and compare its fragrance with that of some of the 'old roses', the 'cabbage roses' (including the *centifolia* species) and the 'damask roses' (the *damascena* species). We also have an abundance of scented spring flowers – such as *Narcissus* and *Hyacinthus* species – and the unique scent of the buds and the leaves of blackcurrant (*Ribes*) species.

Warmer climates also offer an abundance of fragrant flowers – jasmine, freesia, gardenia, tuberose, *Aglaia*, citrus blossoms, cassie (*Acacia farnesiana*), mimosa (*Acacia dealbata*); and you might have access to some tropical blooms, such as frangipani (*Plumeria* species), champaca (*Michelia* species), *Pandanus* species and many more.

Sometimes a visit to a florist can yield some unexpected treasures too…

From the herb garden to the kitchen

In older times, physic gardens would be filled with medicinal herbs, strewing herbs and bee plants. If you do not have access to a herb garden, you can find potted herbs at garden centres and markets. It is well worth taking time to smell the fresh leaves of common culinary herbs – basil and its varieties, bay laurel, coriander, dill, lemon balm, marjoram, mint and its varieties, oregano, parsley, rosemary, sage and its varieties, tarragon, and thyme and its varieties. Once you have familiarised yourself with their aromas, it might be time to move into the kitchen, where the olfactory journey continues!

26

Stimulate Your Senses with an Olfactory Culinary Experience

This is the final phase of resetting the nose, and emphasises the links between our senses of taste and smell. Here, you can prepare dishes and cook with the herbs that you have encountered, and take the time to associate smells with flavours. Remember that we eat with all of our senses, and so take time to notice how herbs and spices can make food visually appealing. You will find that you start to become mindful when eating – and this too is a very good thing! When you use mixtures of herbs – such as the classic bouquet garni, or the parsley/lemon/garlic trio of Spanish cuisine, or lemongrass and chilli in Thai cuisine – can you discern the individual herbs? Lemon and other citrus juices and zests are often used with herbs for flavouring, so include these in your investigations too.

Spices offer another exciting olfactory dimension to food. Culinary spices are usually dried, and benefit from a light dry roasting and grinding to release their aroma (unless, of course, this is accomplished at the beginning of a process or recipe). Here, you really can introduce the aromas of the world into your kitchen. First, make the time to savour the fragrance of individual spices, and then, equipped with some recipes, start cooking and associating aroma with flavour. The list of spices to experience is considerable, but those that are important from both the fragrance and culinary angles are black pepper (and there are many other types of pepper to enjoy), caraway seeds, cardamom, celery seeds, cinnamon bark ('sticks'), clove buds, coriander seeds, cumin seeds, fennel seeds, fenugreek seeds, ginger root, juniperberry, nigella seeds, nutmeg, pimento, saffron, star anise, turmeric and vanilla pods.

This part is entirely up to you; the intention is to help you immerse yourself in your sense of smell on a day-to-day basis. The sensory exercises with essential oils and aromatic extracts can be carried out concurrently.

27

Immerse Yourself in the World of Aromatic Plant Extracts

As we noted earlier, you do not need to work through the aromatics in Part II strictly in the order in which they are presented, nor do you need to experience every one that is mentioned. Simply aim to broaden and share your experience at every opportunity. It has been mentioned several times that you should keep good records. This can be done using a notebook in the style of a diary, and this approach is probably easiest to maintain. However, your olfactory notes can be more structured if you enter your observations on an 'Excel' spreadsheet or similar electronic file. This way you can organise your olfactory experiences as you wish, adding to them as you progress, in a way that is accessible and meaningful to you.

Most important is to be aware of your senses, be mindful, open up to the beautiful realm of fragrance and allow it to become part of you, share it with others and let it enrich your life.

Appendix 1

ODOUR TYPES AND CHARACTERISTICS ENCOUNTERED IN AROMATIC PLANT EXTRACTS

Table compiled from Williams (1980 and 2000), Lawless (2009) and author's observations.

Abbreviations: e.o. – essential oil; abs. – absolute; res – resinoid

Odour type	Associated characteristics	Examples
Anisic: a scent reminiscent of aniseed.	Often sweet or ethereal	Anisic notes can be found in *star anise, tarragon* and *sweet fennel* e.o., also in *tulsi* (*sacred basil*) e.o. and *exotic basil*. They are often conferred by a group of constituents called phenolic ethers.
Balsamic: a vanilla-like scent with a soothing effect, often found in base notes. Sometimes there are resinous or spicy subsidiary notes.	Sweet and/or warm, smooth	Balsamic notes can be found in *benzoin* res., *labdanum* res. and abs., *opopanax* res., *Peru balsam, tolu balsam, vanilla* abs., *cacao* abs.
Camphoraceous: an odour reminiscent of camphor, somewhat medicated, and may have elements of menthol or eucalyptus.	Medicated, pungent, harsh	A typical camphoraceous example is *white camphor* e.o.; however, many others including e.o.s from the 'paperbark trees' have camphoraceous notes such as *niaouli, cajuput* and *tea tree*. Camphoraceous notes are also found in herbal oils such as *spike lavender* e.o. and some *eucalyptus* and *rosemary* oils.
Caramel: a scent reminiscent of burnt sugar, with balsamic characteristics.	Sweet, warm	*Tuberose* abs., although a heavy floral, has subsidiary caramel notes.
Cineolic: eucalyptus-like.	Medicated, diffusive	Most of the 'pharmaceutical' eucalyptus oils are dominated by the constituent 1,8-cineole, an oxide that imparts the characteristic odour.

Odour type	Associated characteristics	Examples
Citrus: the scent of citrus fruit peel. Also, lemony notes fall into this category.	Fresh, light, crisp, sometimes bitter in subsidiary notes. Lemony notes can be sweet and fruity, rosy, or harsh and coarse.	Typical citrus notes are found in the top notes of citrus peel oils – *bergamot, cédrat, combava (kaffir lime) peel, grapefruit, lemon, lime, mandarin, orange* (bitter and sweet), *tangerine.* Lemony notes are found in *Litsea cubeba* e.o. (sweet, fruity); *Eucalyptus citriodora* e.o. and *citronella* e.o. (harsh rosy-lemon); *lemongrass* e.o. (harsh, coarse); *lemon verbena* e.o., *petitgrain combava* (kaffir lime leaf) e.o. and top notes of *ginger* e.o.
Coniferous: the fragrance of coniferous trees, their needles, resins and cones and berries; subsidiary camphoraceous, green and resinous notes.	Fresh, invigorating, but can be perceived as disinfectant-like because of associations with this particular application.	The coniferous trees all share this note – but most notably the *fir, spruce* and *pine* e.o.s. The disinfectant-like note is imparted by the constituents α- and β-pinene. *Atlas cedar* is warm and camphoraceous with soft floral notes, while *Virginian cedar* is mild, dry, and woody/balsamic. *Cypress* and *juniper* are more resinous.
Earthy: the smell of damp soil; fresh, but with a vegetation/fungal nuance.	'Rich', 'damp', 'musty' are adjectives that can be applied.	Several e.o.s have earthy characteristics, including *spikenard, patchouli* and *vetiver.*
Faecal: the smell of excrement.	Although in its unadulterated form this provokes disgust, traces may be found in some e.o.s and abs.	Trace amounts of faecal-smelling compounds can be found in some of the 'indolic' floral oils such as *jasmine* abs., *orange flower* abs. and *white champaca* abs., giving a 'natural' element to the odour profile.

Floral: suggestive of flowers, either a single flower or a bouquet. Subsidiary types include rosy, indolic (white blooms), jasmine-like, tropical, hyacinth, lily-like, violet-like. Subsidiary notes include green, fruity, spicy, citrus, herbal, caramel, honey, waxy.	As the category is so wide, many adjectives are used to describe floral characteristics. These include sweet, soft, rich, intense, heady, heavy, light, delicate, fresh.	Rosy: *rose otto* e.o. and *rose* abs., *rose geranium* e.o. and abs. Indolic: *jasmine* abs., *jasmine sambac* abs., *neroli* e.o. and *orange blossom* absolute, *tuberose* abs., *white chamapaca* abs. Tropical: *ylang ylang* e.o., *red champaca* (fruity floral), *tiaré* abs., *frangipani* abs. Violet-like: *violet flower* abs., *orris root* (also floral, woody).
Fruity: a sense of edible fruits, and not restricted to citrus. Subsidiary types include dried fruit, raisin, pear, plum and apple.	Sweet, sour, sharp, smooth, mellow, fresh	Fruity notes can be detected in *jasmine* abs., *frangipani* abs., *tagetes* e.o., *lavender* e.o., *clove bud* e.o. Dried fruit, raisin and plum notes are in the floral *osmanthus* abs. Apple-like notes are in *Roman chamomile* e.o. and *tagetes* e.o. *Blackcurrant bud* abs. is fruity but with dominant green notes and a 'catty' element.
Green: reminiscent of crushed green leaves, fresh peas in the pod, cucumber, cut green bell peppers.	Fresh, cool, light, sharp	*Violet leaf* abs. is typical; so are *galbanum* e.o. and res. (also musty, earthy notes). Green notes are also in many herbal oils, especially *mint* e.o.s. *Geranium* e.o. and abs. are floral/rose with green/minty subsidiary notes.

Odour type	Associated characteristics	Examples
Hay: the scent of hay drying in the sun, reminiscent of the countryside; typical of the agrestic family. Subsidiary notes include coconut, green.	Warm, mellow, sweet	The hay note is imparted by a constituent of grass, clover and tonka beans – *coumarin* (a synthetic version) is available in perfumery. *Hay* abs. is typical. *Tonka bean* abs. is balsamic (vanilla) with hay notes. *Lavender, immortelle, genet* and *oakmoss* absolutes have subsidiary hay notes.
Herbaceous: the scent of aromatic culinary and medicinal herbs. Subsidiary notes often include green and woody, sometimes floral, minty, anisic or tabac.	Sharp, pungent, penetrating, fresh, light	*Sage* e.o. and abs., *thyme* e.o. and abs., *artemisia* e.o. and abs., *clary sage* e.o. and abs., *rosemary, marjoram* and *lavender* e.o.s are typical herbaceous scents. *Rosemary* and *marjoram* e.o.s are fresh, pungent. *Lavender* e.o. is light herbaceous with floral and woody notes. *Thyme* abs. and *clary sage* e.o. have warm subsidiary tabac notes. *Lemon myrtle* has a lemon subsidiary note. *Laurel* abs. is herbaceous with green and anisic subsidiary notes, as is *basil* e.o.
Honey: a sweet odour reminiscent of honey; may have floral undertones.	Sweet, smooth	In perfumery honey notes are derived from *beeswax* abs., which is sweet, smooth and honeyed, and also waxy. Subsidiary honey notes can be detected in some florals, such as *tuberose* abs., *white ginger lily* abs., *linden blossom* abs. and *immortelle* abs.

Medicated: odours associated with traditional external medications; includes camphoraceous, minty, wintergreen, cineolic, terpenic and thymolic odours.	Penetrating, diffusive, pungent, 'warming' or 'cooling' by association	*White camphor* e.o is camphoraceous; often the camphoraceous note is considered to be warming. By contrast, the minty note is cooling. *Eucalyptus globulus* is cineolic, *juniper berry* e.o. is terpenic, *thyme* e.o. is thymolic. The *wintergreen* note is given by an aromatic ester – methyl salicylate.
Minty: the odour of mint. Green, herbaceous and minty subsidiary notes are often present.	Fresh, penetrating, sharp, refreshing, light	*Spearmint* and *peppermint* e.o.s are typical, with sharp and penetrating characteristics. *Mint* abs. may have a smoother quality. Minty notes are also found in herbal oils such as *pennyroyal* e.o. and florals such as *geranium* abs.
Mossy: reminiscent of the forest floor and its vegetation. Green, fungal, earthy and woody notes can be present too.	Deep, rich, natural	The botanical sources are *lichens* (a symbiotic association between an alga and a fungus) that grow on the bark of oak trees and conifers, yielding oakmoss and treemoss absolutes – the archetypal mossy scent of perfumery essential in chypre and fougère ('fern') fragrances.
Oily: this is often accompanied by the word 'fatty', although there are subtle differences. An oily note is reminiscent of fixed vegetable oils such as linseed.	Faint, not dominant	Oily notes are present in *lemongrass* e.o. and *Atlas cedar* e.o., while fatty notes (smoother and with more body) can be detected in *jasmine* abs.
Peppery: reminiscent of freshly ground black pepper; a woody/spicy odour.	Warm, dry (opposite of sweet), fresh	*Black pepper* e.o. is typical. Peppery, almost effervescent notes are also present in the citrus oil of *bergamot*; this effect possibly conferred by the shared constituent terpinen-4-ol. *Coriander seed* e.o. also has peppery notes.

Odour type	Associated characteristics	Examples
Resinous: the scent of tree resins and exudates. Subsidiary notes include balsamic and coniferous.	Fresh, sweet, clean	*Frankincense* e.o. is resinous, with a typical coniferous pine-like note and fresh lemon notes in the top note. *Myrrh* is resinous but also balsamic, sweet, spicy and somewhat medicated. *Benzoin* resinoid is typically balsamic, yet has a resinous quality. *Juniper berry* e.o. is coniferous, sweet, fresh and resinous, without the pine disinfectant note. Most of the conifers have resinous notes.
Rosy: a scent reminiscent of roses, but not necessarily sourced from the rose. Subsidiary notes are floral, herbal, green, spicy and woody.	Sweet, light, mild, rich	*Rose otto* (e.o.) is typical; this has waxy top notes. Other rosy-scented aromatics are *geranium* (green, rosy), *palmarosa* (a scented grass with rosy herbal notes), *immortelle* (rich, sweet, rosy, honey), *rosewood* (floral, rosy, woody and mild) and *guaiacwood* (woody, smooth, mild, balsamic).
Smoky: the odour of smouldering woods and leaves, when smelled from a distance.	Deep, fragrant	*Cypress* e.o. is woody, resinous and balsamic with smoky notes. *Vetiver* e.o. is earthy, woody, rooty and green, with smoky undertones.
Spicy: the scents of aromatic culinary spices. Sometimes woody subsidiary notes.	Pungent, warm, dry, sweet – although there is enormous variety in the spicy characteristics (see the examples opposite)	*Caraway seed* (sweet), *cardamom* (cineolic top), *cinnamon bark and leaf* (strong, sweet, warm, floral or fruity notes), *clove bud* (fruity, woody), *coriander seed* (light, woody), *ginger* (lemony, warm, woody, pungent), *nutmeg* (warm, pine-like, ethereal), *pimento berry* (sweet, warm, clove-like, herbaceous), *turmeric* (fresh, spicy, woody).

Tabac: the odour of semi-dried pipe tobacco. Subsidiary notes include hay and green nuances.	Sweet, pungent, rich, warm	*Tobacco leaf* abs. is typical. Also detected in the dry oil notes of *German chamomile* e.o. and the middle notes of *clary sage* e.o.
Waxy: a note reminiscent of paraffin wax or beeswax. Usually a subsidiary note.	Soft, rich, warm	*Beeswax* abs. has a waxy note, and this is also found in the dryout of *jasmine* abs. and the top note of *rose otto*.
Wintergreen: the medicated scent of wintergreen oil.	Strong, penetrating, diffusive	*Wintergreen* e.o. is typical, as is *sweet birch* e.o. The medicated scent is conferred by the main constituent, methyl salicylate. This is present in much smaller amounts in the intensely floral, diffusive ylang ylang; however, you can still detect the medicated wintergreen note.
Woody: the scent of the woods of exotic trees. Balsamic, resinous, floral and camphoraceous are possible subsidiary notes in this category. Many spice and root oils have a woody note.	The woody category has many associated adjectives – soft, mild, sweet	Arguably the most important woody oil is that of *true sandalwood* (soft, sweet and warm; some will detect a faint urinous note). *Guaiacwood* and *rosewood* are sweet, balsamic and mild and have floral/rosy notes.

Appendix 2

SOME NOTES ON CHEMISTRY

Volatile oils and their extraction
The scent of aromatic plants is due to the presence of volatile oils which contain secondary metabolites – plant constituents that are not involved in growth or development, but have other complex biological and ecological roles, many of which have yet to be defined. Plant volatile oils are found in specialised cells which are located in various anatomical parts of plants. Frequently they are located in the flowers, but they may also be found in leaves, bark, fruit and seeds; also in woody parts such as stems and roots (Williams 1996). These oils can be extracted by physical means, such as expression in the case of citrus peel, maceration in oils or fats, and water or steam distillation to yield essential oils. Solvent extraction yields aromatic products known as concretes and absolutes, and this is widely used for the extraction of floral oils such as jasmine. Sometimes ultrasonic extraction precedes solvent extraction – this disrupts the cells, releasing the volatile oils, and thus helps the efficiency of the extraction process. Recent developments in extraction technology are vacuum microwave hydro-distillation (VMHD), which produces essential oils that have not been subjected to thermal degradation, and supercritical fluid extraction (SFE), which produces volatiles very similar to the ones in the plant, because the solvent (usually carbon dioxide) has a near ambient critical temperature of 31°C, thus preventing heat and chemical modifications in the product (Tonutti and Liddle 2010).

The big picture
Volatile oils are chemically complex; however, generally, the constituents fall into two large categories – the *terpenoids* and the *phenyl propanoids*. These are all based on structures of carbon and hydrogen atoms – and they belong to the massive class of chemicals called *hydrocarbons*. Generally, the terpenes and terpenoids are composed of chains, cyclic structures, or cycles with short chains, and even some 'bridged' carbon frames, while the phenylpropanoids are characterised by the presence of a specific type of ring structure, known as an 'aromatic' or 'benzene' ring. These terpenes and phenyl propane-type molecules are the parent chemicals of a huge variety of other molecules – known as their derivatives – which include at least one oxygen atom in their structure, and so are sometimes called oxygenated derivatives. Some of these

derivatives are, in turn, the starting point for other chemicals to be formed. So we do have a very complicated picture. Here the intention is simply to give an overview of some of the more common constituents and relate these to their odours.

The two large classes of constituents, the terpenoids and phenylpropanoids, are defined by the biochemical pathway in which they are formed within the plant, and each is comprised of smaller classes of constituents. These smaller classes are defined by similarities in the molecular make-up of their members. In chemistry and biology there is a general rule that structure determines function. In other words, and to make this relevant to us, the structure of these molecules (i.e. the component atoms and their arrangement, including they type of the bonds that hold the atoms together) is directly related to the way that each molecule will behave, its chemical properties, its therapeutic or hazardous potential, and, of course, the way it smells.

Terpenes and terpenoids

The terpenes and their derivatives, the terpenoids, are named after turpentine, which gives a clue to the origins of some of them. The *pinenes* found in many conifers are monoterpenes (molecules which contain 10 carbon atoms) with a characteristic fresh, piney, coniferous smell. You will sometimes see a prefix, α- (alpha) or β- (beta) pinene. This indicates that the constituent exists in two forms, known as isomers. Their molecules are made up of exactly the same atoms, but in a subtly different configuration; for example, in the case of α- and β-pinene a double bond is located in a different position. Other monoterpenes include *limonene*, with a dull citrus odour, found in citrus peel oils. You will sometimes see a *d-* or *l-* prefix, and, again, this is indicative of isomerism – in this case it is optical isomerism, where the molecule of one form is the mirror image of the other form, rather like looking at your right and left hands. Often optical isomers have different odours. Staying with the limonene example, the *d-* isomer that predominates in many citrus oils has a weak, citrus/lemony scent, while the *l-* isomer smells more like turpentine. Monoterpenes often are found in the top notes of citrus and pine oils.

Larger terpene molecules (with 15 carbon atoms) are the *sesquiterpenes*, and as these molecules are bigger, they are heavier and do not evaporate as quickly as the monoterpenes; they are often found in base notes. Many of their names reflect their botanical sources, such as the *santalenes* (here we find α- and β- isomers) in sandalwood, or *zingiberene* in ginger.

The *terpenoids* are formed in the plant from their parent constituents – the monoterpenes or sesquiterpenes. Because of the presence of oxygen atoms in the molecules, they are known as oxygenated derivatives – and they dominate essential oil chemistry. The oxygen atom is part of small groups of atoms on a molecule; these groups are known as 'functional groups', and are important in not only the classification but also the properties of the constituent. The monoterpenoids include the *alcohols* such as the light, mild, floral-woody scented *d-linalool* which is in many oils including lavender, and the sweet rosy *geraniol* in geranium. *Citral*[1] belongs to the group of constituents known as *aldehydes*; it has a harsh lemon odour and is found in lemongrass, while *citronellal*, with its citrus and rosy odour, is found in litsea and lemon-scented eucalyptus. *Ketones* are yet another group of terpenoids. *Menthone* is the penetrating, cooling, minty ketone in peppermint; *l-carvone* also has a minty odour and is found in spearmint, while its isomer *d-carvone* has a caraway-like scent and is found in caraway seed oil. *Esters* are also derived from the terpenes. Examples are the herbal, fruity, apple-like esters in Roman chamomile; the well-investigated *linalyl acetate* (derived from linalool) with its fresh, light, herbal, fruity scent dominates true lavender, clary sage and bergamot oils, and *geranyl acetate* (derived from geraniol) has a sweet, rosy, fruity aroma.

The sesquiterpenoids include alcohols such as the mild and woody α- and β-*santalols* in sandalwood, the faint woody *cedrol* in Virginian cedar, and the herbal, patchouli-like *patchoulol* in patchouli – these constituents are all significantly related to the aromas of their volatile oils.

Phenylpropanoids

The *phenylpropanoids* are synthesised in a different biochemical pathway. This is a diverse group, but all the molecules share a distinguishing feature – the presence of an 'aromatic ring' structure. Although phenylpropanoids are not as numerous as the terpenes, they do have interesting odours and characteristics. Here we have the spicy, clove-like *eugenol* (a *phenol*) in clove oil, the pleasant floral rose/hyacinth scented *phenylethanol* (an *aromatic alcohol*) in rose, and the sweet, ethereal, *trans-anethole*[2] (a *phenolic ether*) in sweet fennel and star anise. There are also many *aromatic esters*, found in floral oils such as jasmine and tuberose, and the medicated *methyl salicylate* of wintergreen oil; and *aldehydes* such as *cinnamaldehyde* in cinnamon, and *vanillin* in benzoin and vanilla.

Very occasionally occurring, but nonetheless important from the odour perspective, there are nitrogen-containing compounds such as *pyrazines*, which give the intense green notes in galbanum oil, and the *anthranilates*, which can give floral/fruity or fishy notes in mandarin oil. Sulphur-containing compounds (*thioles*) are present in some oils – such as garlic

---

1 To complicate matters, citral is in fact the name given to a naturally occurring mixture of two aldehydes – neral and geranial!

2 The prefix *trans-* indicates another type of isomerism known as geometrical isomerism; *cis*-isomers have groups of similar atoms on one side of a double bond; *trans*-isomers have the same groups of atoms on the opposite sides of a double bond. Examples are geraniol (*cis*-) and nerol (*trans*-).

and onion – which have extremely powerful, diffusive and pungent odours, rendering them unsuitable for perfumery but useful in flavouring; they are also antiseptics. Blackcurrant bud absolute contains traces of a thiole named *4-methoxy-2-methylbutan-2-thiol*, which has a very low detection threshold of 1 in 1,000,000 billion!

Appendix 3

BUILDING ACCORDS

Preparatory notes

Here, ratios are *not* given. The accords are simple – pairs (duos), trios and quartets – and can be used as 'building blocks' to create more complex accords. Experimenting is part of the learning process, and it is not the intention here to be overly prescriptive. Begin by preparing blotters and holding these together to gain an impression of the combinations, or adding a few drops to one blotter.

You can also prepare dilutions in an odourless vegetable base, such as jojoba. This will allow you to use some of the very powerful aromatics in sufficient dilution, so that they are more pleasant and more representative of their natural counterparts. These can be used as simple perfumes, *but*, before applying them to the skin, check safety aspects, because some aromatic extracts are phototoxic (cause burning when applied to skin prior to exposure to sunlight), and others are irritant or sensitising (can cause an allergic skin reaction). So exercise common sense and caution. Some of the resinoids may feel quite sticky and are not so suitable for application on the skin.

To prepare a blend in jojoba

First, work out your blend on paper – compose your base, middle and top accords, ensuring that your blend will be cohesive by considering the bridges within the accords and between them. For an oil-based blend, you might like to work with a top: middle: base ratio of 1:1:1, because the fixed oil delays evaporation.

You will need a graduated glass beaker (20ml capacity), glass droppers, a 15ml bottle with dropper insert and cap, a glass rod for stirring, and a label for the bottle. It might also be necessary to warm some of the paste-like absolutes so that they are easier to handle, and the tip of the glass rod can be used to dispense a 'drop'.

By volume: To make an approximate 10 per cent concentration, you will need to add approximately 30 drops of aromatic extracts and then make up to 15ml with jojoba. First add the ingredients of your base accord, up to 10 drops. Mix and smell as you go. Then add the middle notes (again, 10 drops), sampling and making notes as you progress, because there is always room for adjustment. Finally, the top notes (10 drops) should be added. Again, smell carefully as your fragrance is being created. Every single drop will alter the scent! Focus, use your olfactory awareness, and let the experience enter your memory. Because measuring in drops is not very accurate, there is some room for manoeuvre without altering the concentration significantly – so you can adjust your blend by adding a few more drops of your selected oils (up to 5 drops), or even introducing a new element if you feel so inclined. It is all about perception and learning, it is part of the journey, and *don't forget to write down exactly what is in the blend, for future reference...*

If you do decide to make aromatic blends, you will find that they change and 'mature' over time. They should keep quite well if stored in dark glass bottles and in a cool place. Jojoba is suggested as the base because it is quite resistant to oxidation – it has good keeping qualities, unlike some other vegetable oils.

Some simple accords (duos, trios and quartets)
Bergamot e.o. and coriander seed e.o.
Carrot seed e.o. and coriander seed e.o.
Clove bud e.o. and rose abs.
Galbanum e.o., blackcurrant bud abs., Roman chamomile e.o.
Galbanum e.o., blackcurrant bud abs., hyacinth abs.
Hay abs., vanilla abs., tobacco abs., cacao abs.
Jasmine abs. and caraway seed e.o.
Jasmine abs. and celery seed e.o.
Jasmine abs., rose abs., cedarwood e.o.
Labdanum res. and jasmine abs.
Linden blossom abs. and lime e.o.
Mimosa abs., blackcurrant bud abs., cacao abs.
Patchouli e.o. and rose abs.
Patchouli e.o. and jasmine abs.
Sandalwood e.o. and rose abs.
Sandalwood e.o. and jasmine abs.
Sandalwood e.o. and white champaca abs.
Tuberose abs. and celery seed e.o.
Tuberose abs. and cumin seed e.o.
Vanilla abs. and rose abs.
Ylang ylang extra e.o. or abs., bergamot e.o., lemon e.o., galbanum e.o.

Some base accords (simple trios and quartets)
Benzoin res., sandalwood e.o., tolu balsam
Benzoin res., black pepper e.o. (carries to top note), pimento e.o.
Benzoin res., myrrh abs., sandalwood e.o., vetiver e.o.

Hay abs., labdanum res., opopanax res.

Hay abs., lavender abs., tobacco leaf abs.

Labdanum res., vanilla abs., frankincense e.o. (an 'ambra' effect)

Labdanum res., vetiver e.o., benzoin res.

Oakmoss abs., sandalwood e.o., patchouli e.o. (a 'chypre' base, for a floral heart and bergamot top)

Patchouli e.o., sandalwood e.o., labdanum res.

Tolu balsam res., vanilla abs., opopanax res.

Vanilla abs., sandalwood e.o., patchouli e.o., cacao abs. (rich balsamic/woody/earthy)

Vanilla abs., tolu balsam res., sandalwood e.o.

Vetiver e.o., tobacco leaf abs., patchouli e.o.

Heart accords (simple trios and quartets)

Red or white champaca abs., jasmine abs., nutmeg e.o.

Clary sage abs., clove bud e.o., jasmine abs.

Clary sage abs., lavender abs., laurel leaf abs.

Clary sage abs., Roman chamomile abs. or e.o., blackcurrant bud abs.

Frangipani abs., rose abs., clove bud e.o.

Frangipani abs., jasmine abs., ylang ylang extra abs. or e.o.

Frangipani abs., ylang ylang extra abs. or e.o., nutmeg e.o.

Genet abs., hay abs., blackcurrant bud abs.

Guaiacwood e.o., rose abs., violet leaf abs.

Jasmine abs., caraway seed e.o., ylang ylang extra abs. or e.o.

Jasmine sambac abs., white champaca abs., celery seed e.o.

Jasmine abs., cardamom e.o., frankincense e.o.

Jasmine abs., ylang ylang extra abs. or e.o., aglaia abs.

Laurel leaf abs., lavender abs., thyme abs.

Lavender abs., thyme abs., clary sage abs., rose abs.

Lavender abs., thyme abs., violet leaf abs.

Mimosa abs., jasmine abs., orange blossom abs., ylang ylang extra abs. or e.o.

Mimosa abs., violet leaf abs., blackcurrant bud abs.

Orange blossom abs., tuberose abs., white champaca abs.

Osmanthus abs., mimosa abs., aglaia abs.

Pink lotus abs., mimosa abs., linden abs.

Pink lotus abs., jasmine abs., orange blossom abs.

Pink lotus abs., rose abs., violet leaf abs.

Roman chamomile abs., lavender abs., rose abs.

Rose abs., jasmine abs., ylang ylang extra abs. or e.o.

Rose abs., geranium e.o., ylang ylang extra e.o., clove bud e.o.

Tuberose abs., caraway abs., jasmine abs., orange blossom abs.

Top accords (simple trios and quartets)

Bergamot e.o., carrot seed e.o., coriander seed e.o., rose otto

Bergamot e.o., petitgrain e.o., rose otto

Bergamot e.o., coriander seed e.o., petitgrain e.o., mimosa abs.

Bergamot e.o., basil e.o., coriander seed e.o., petitgrain e.o., rose otto

Bergamot e.o., rosewood e.o., bitter orange e.o.

Bergamot e.o., mandarin e.o., petitgrain e.o., rosewood e.o.

Bergamot e.o., cédrat e.o., mimosa abs.

Bitter orange e.o., mandarin e.o., lime e.o.

Caraway seed e.o., celery seed e.o., coriander seed e.o., bergamot e.o.

Coriander seed e.o., carrot seed e.o., yellow grapefruit e.o., black pepper e.o.

Fir e.o., Virginian cedar e.o., lavender e.o., pine e.o.

Petitgrain e.o., bitter orange e.o., neroli e.o., rose otto

Rose otto, black pepper e.o., galbanum e.o.

Virginian cedar e.o., rosewood e.o., coriander seed e.o., bergamot e.o.

GLOSSARY

Absolute: A highly concentrated aromatic extract obtained by alcoholic extraction of the concrete, which is obtained by the process of solvent extraction (or enfleurage) of aromatic plant material.

Accord: In perfumery, a combination of aromatics that combine to give a particular fragrance effect.

Agrestic: An odour that is reminiscent of the countryside.

Amber: A perfume note that is powdery and reminiscent of vanilla.

Ambergris: A pathological secretion that occurs in just one per cent of adult male sperm whales. If it is expelled by the whale and floats in the sea, eventually water, air and sunlight transform malodorous matter into a rare and costly perfume material, which is washed up on the shore.

Amygdala: An almond-shaped structure that is located deep within the centre of the limbic system of the brain; associated with basic survival and emotions such as anger and fear. The amygdala is larger in male brains than female.

Animalic: An odour reminiscent of an animal source – musk, castoreum, civet. A plant aromatic with an animalic odour is ambrette seed; this is often used as a botanical musk substitute.

Aromachemical: An odorous chemical, which is used in the flavour and fragrance industry.

Aromatic: This can mean two things – either describing a substance that has an odour (usually pleasant), or with reference to a molecule that has a 'benzene ring' as part of its structure. For example, an 'aromatic aldehyde' is a molecule with an aldehyde functional group (a small group of carbon and oxygen atoms arranged in a way that defines the molecule with the specific structure and properties of the chemical family known as aldehydes) attached to an aromatic ring structure.

Base note: An aromatic of relatively low volatility, or an odour that persists after the top and middle notes have evaporated; usually given by constituents with low volatility. Also refers to the dryout note, or the drydown.

Beeswax absolute: A rich, warm, honey- and hay-like extract of honeycombed beeswax.

Blotter: A thick, absorbent strip of paper or card, used to sample liquid aromatic extracts; the blotter or 'smelling strip' allows an even and unhindered evaporation of the volatile constituents, giving an accurate impression of the odour over a period of time.

Body note: Also known as the middle note, this is the sensory impact of the moderately volatile constituents of an aromatic material or a perfume, with traces of the top notes and the emergence of the base notes becoming apparent; intermediate lasting power.

Brain stem: Connects the cerebrum to the spinal cord; it consists of the midbrain (where the two hemispheres come together), the pons varolii (a bridge of connecting fibres) and the medulla oblongata (continuous with the spinal cord). All three parts are vital for survival, and control the heart, the blood vessels and breathing. There are also reflex centres in the medulla oblongata – for sneezing and vomiting if something is irritating the respiratory tract or stomach.

Camphor: Natural camphor is referred to as *d*-camphor because it is optically active – it will bend a beam of polarised light to the right. (The *d*- stands for *dextro*-rotatory.) Synthetic camphor, or camphor derived from fractional distillation of petroleum, is a fraction of the cost, but it is not optically active. It can also be obtained from pinene, converted to camphene and then treated with acetic acid and nitrobenzene to form camphor.

Castoreum: The beaver has glands under its tail which secrete oil that waterproofs its coat to prevent waterlogging. Castoreum is the dried secretion of these glands; an absolute and tincture are used in perfumery. The tincture has a tenacious, leather-like, phenolic odour that is often used in leather and tabac masculine fragrances.

Cerebrum: The largest brain structure, which surrounds most of the other structures; it is divided into two sides (hemispheres), which are separated by a deep groove running from the back of the brain to the forehead. The two hemispheres are connected by the corpus callosum. Each is divided by fissures into four lobes – the frontal, temporal, parietal and occipital. The functions of the cerebrum ('grey matter') are to initiate and control movement, and to receive impulses from our sensory organs.

Chypre: François Coty created the first modern chypre fragrance in 1917. It is a perfume type containing a base accord of oakmoss, labdanum, sandalwood and musk (and often including patchouli and clary sage) and a floral heart (often rose and jasmine), with a bergamot top note.

Cineolic: A penetrating, eucalyptus-like odour, which gets its name from one of the principal chemical components of eucalyptus oil: 1,8-cineole.

Cis- and trans-isomerism: A type of geometrical isomerism; *cis*-isomers have groups of similar atoms on one side of a double bond; *trans*-isomers have the same groups of atoms on the opposite sides of a double bond. An example is geraniol (*cis*-) and nerol (*trans*-).

Civet: The glandular secretion of the civet, *Viverra civetta* and other *Viverra* species, small animals related to the weasel. In its raw form it has a pungent, repellent, faecal odour. A tincture is made from the secretion of the abdominal glands for use in perfumery; this is sweet and reminiscent of animal fur, and used to impart lift to chypre and delicate floral perfumes. The main constituents are civettone and skatole.

Concrete: An aromatic solid or semi-solid extract containing essential oil, waxes and pigments, obtained by solvent extraction of aromatic plant material.

Corpus callosum: The structure ('white matter') that separates and connects the right and left hemispheres of the cerebrum. It is composed of long neuron branches, and is larger in female brains than male.

Cross-modal: A term used to denote an interrelationship across the senses; for example, smells may have associations with tastes and flavours, foods, sounds, music, words, images, shapes, colours, textures, etc.

Deterpenated: Refers to an essential oil that has been rectified to remove the terpene component; often has a more pleasant scent, and is less likely to present solubility problems when incorporated into scented products.

Diffusive: A characteristic of some fragrance compounds, essential oils and absolutes where the scent rapidly permeates the atmosphere.

Dryout: The odour that remains when an aromatic material is in the very final stages of evaporation.

Enfleurage: The process of absorbing the fragrance from fresh flowers of a single species into a purified fatty medium over a period of time, to produce a *pomade*.

Essential oil: A volatile product obtained by a physical process from a natural source of a single botanical species, which corresponds to that species in name and odour.

Evaporation: The change in physical state from liquid to gas/vapour.

Extra: The first fraction of the distillation process of ylang ylang is denoted 'extra'; ylang ylang extra is considered to have a superior aroma to the subsequent fractions, which are known as No. 1, 2 and 3.

Extract: The soluble matter obtained from an aromatic plant by washing with a solvent that is then recovered by vacuum distillation. Extracts include concretes, absolutes and resinoids.

Extrait: The French word for 'extract'. Originally, extrait perfumes were produced by alcoholic extraction of enfleurage pomade (see entry 'enfleurage'). Early extraits were of the floral type, such as rose, jasmine, tuberose, cassie, violet, jonquil, bitter orange blossom and mignonette. The term came to denote strong alcoholic solutions of perfume compound (or essence), and it is currently used to mean the strongest form of alcoholic perfume that is commercially available (between 5 and 20% of perfume compound in strong ethanol).

Expression: A mechanical process of scarification and compression for obtaining the volatile oil from the flavedo of citrus fruits; cold-expression is considered to yield the best-quality oils.

Exudate: A resinous substance produced by the cambium of some woody plants; aromatic exudates include benzoin, frankincense and myrrh.

Fixative: A perfume ingredient that can prolong the lasting power of the main theme of a fragrance.

Foin: Foin absolute is obtained from the sweet-scented vernal grass (*Anthoxanthum odoratum*) by solvent extraction; the distilled product is known as flouve essential oil.

Fougère: A perfume type, literally 'fern', usually containing coumarin (a hay-scented aromachemical) and lavender oil; derived from the scented soap *Fougère Royale* (Houbigant 1882).

Frontal lobes (cortex): Located at the front of the cerebrum behind the frontal bone (forehead), this is thought to be the most recently evolved part of the human brain. This is where we organise our response to complex problems, plan, construct and adapt strategies, and search our memory to support our decisions. It is also where socially appropriate and productive behaviour is managed; it is where, for example, facial expressions and non-verbal behaviours are interpreted and our responses managed. The posterior part of the frontal lobes is concerned with movement – the 'motor areas'.

γ- (gamma): A prefix on some constituent names, indicating positional isomerism, such as γ-terpinene and γ-decalactone.

Geosmin: An organic chemical – a bicyclic alcohol – responsible for the earthy taste and smell of beets, also for the smell in the air after rain has fallen on dry ground.

Hawthorn: *Cratageus oxycantha* of the Rosaceae family is the common hedge tree of Europe, whose blossoms have a sweet, heady scent. In perfumery, anisic aldehyde is used to recall this odour type.

Hippocampus: Located deep in the brain, the hippocampus processes new memories for storage. The hippocampus is affected in some diseases such as Alzheimer's disease.

Hypothalamus: Located at the base of the brain in the deep layers of the cerebral cortex, where the brain and hormonal systems interact, the hypothalamus maintains a state of homeostasis (balance), monitoring bodily functions such as blood pressure and temperature, and controlling appetite and weight.

Immunoglobulins: Antibodies produced by white blood cells that are important in our immune response; broadly speaking, IgE – allergic reactions, IgG – phacocytosis (engulfing and removal of invading microorganisms), IgA – neutralising activities (e.g. preventing pathogens from attaching to and penetrating tissues) and IgM – the first antibodies released during the immune response.

Isomer: One of two or more compounds where the molecular formula is identical, but the atoms are arranged differently; for example, α- and β-pinenes are identical apart from the position of a double bond, γ-terpinene is isomeric with α- and β-terpinenes. *Cis*- and *trans*-isomerism is a type of geometrical isomerism; *cis*-isomers have groups of similar atoms on one side of a double bond, *trans*-isomers have the same groups of atoms on the opposite sides of a double bond. An example is geraniol (*cis*-) and nerol (*trans*-). Optical isomerism describes the type of isomerism where the molecule of one form is the mirror image of the other form; for example, *d*- and *l*-limonene, and *d*- and *l*-carvone.

Maceration: The process of soaking a known weight of matter in a known volume of solvent such as a vegetable oil, in a closed vessel, over a given period of time, after which the suspension is filtered, the soluble portion of the matter having dissolved in the solvent. This solution may be standardised to a given strength. If the solvent is alcohol, the resultant liquid is known as a tincture.

Medicated (or 'medicinal'): A term used to describe a scent that is reminiscent of the penetrating smell of some traditional liniments for exterior use; camphor and wintergreen are examples.

Mentholic: The descriptive term for the odour of menthol; related to but distinct from mint.

Middle note: A scent impression given by constituents of intermediate volatility, and often the main contributor to the 'heart', or main theme of a fragrance.

Mignonette: The flowers of *Reseda odorata*, indigenous to Egypt and the Mediterranean. The absolute has an odour reminiscent of violet leaves.

Musk: The abdominal glands of the male musk deer of the Himalayas, Tibet and North India contain a secretion that can be made into a tincture for use in perfumery, although most perfumery musks are now synthetic. The tincture has a radiant, sweet, fresh odour with fruity notes.

Narcotic: In perfumery this word is used to mean a heavy, sleep-inducing scent.

Natural killer cells: Cells that develop in the bone marrow and are also found in the lymph nodes, spleen, tonsils and thymus; they are an important part of our immune response, involved in the early defence against viral infections.

Occipital lobes: Located to the posterior and lying under the occipital bone, this is where visual data is interpreted and routed to other parts of the brain for identification and storage.

Odorant: A substance that possesses an odour.

Oleo-gum resin: A plant exudate composed of water-soluble gum, resin and volatile oil.

Oleoresin: A plant exudate consisting of resin and volatile oil.

Optical isomerism: Where the molecule of one form is the mirror image of the other form; for example, *d*- and *l*-limonenes and *d*- and *l*-carvones. This could be visualised as right- and left-handed versions. The prefixes *d*- and *l*- relate to the phenomenon of optical rotation. Most essential oils show optical activity. One of a pair of optical isomers will rotate a plane of polarised light in a clockwise direction (dextrorotatory) and the other in an anti-clockwise direction (laevorotatory).

Parietal lobes: Located under the parietal bones, lying posterior to the frontal cortex, the parietal lobes receive and process sensory information related to movement and taste.

Phenylethanol: 2-phenylethyl alcohol is the main commercial alcohol apart from ethyl alcohol, and the most used fragrance in the perfumes and cosmetics industry. It is a minor constituent in narcissus, hyacinth, geranium Bourbon, and *Alep* pine, rose and jasmine flowers; up to 60 per cent in rose absolute. It has a sweet, honey, rose-like aroma.

Pomade: A product of the enfleurage process – a fragrance-saturated fat.

Prefrontal cortex: Located in the frontal lobes, this is where our higher cognitive functions occur, such as making 'executive' decisions, planning, and orchestrating our thoughts, actions and social interactions; it is sometimes said to be associated with positive emotion.

Rectified: Some essential oils are subjected to rectification – a process of re-distillation to eliminate unwanted constituents, or to standardise the product.

Resinoid: The product of solvent extraction of an oleo-gum resin or an oleoresin, which contains the odorous constituents.

Sensitisation reaction: Contact sensitisation is an allergic reaction to an antigen that manifests as itching and inflammation. Skin sensitisation is a delayed type of humoural response that is mediated by T-cells.

Solvent: A liquid substance into which another substance can dissolve.

Solvent extraction: The separation of soluble matter from a natural source of plant material, oleo-gum resin or oleoresin, using a pure, volatile solvent. At the end of the process the solvent is recovered by vacuum distillation, leaving behind the product containing the odorous portion of the material. The product is a concrete, which can be further treated to produce an absolute or a resinoid, which in some cases may be distilled to produce a volatile oil.

Steam distillation: A process of distillation in which steam, under pressure, is used to heat a charge in a still, and release and vaporise the volatile molecules. The volatile portion is then condensed back into liquid form and collected in a receiver vessel.

Styrax (storax): Obtained from the tree *Liquidambar orientalis*; a gum with a sweet balsamic scent that exudes from the heartwood if the bark is injured.

Tabac: A fragrance type characterised by the sweet, pungent, warm aroma of cured, semi-dried pipe tobacco.

Temporal lobes: Part of the cerebrum, located behind the temporal bones, responsible for hearing and also smell. This is where memories and emotions are stored; the left lobe is associated with language.

Thalamus: Located at the top of the brain stem, this sorts, processes and directs signals from the spinal cord and the mid-brain up to the cerebrum, and from the cerebrum down to the spinal cord and nervous system.

Top note: The immediate impact of an aromatic material or fragrance, given by its most volatile constituents and some of the slightly less volatile ones; sometimes fleeting, or lacking in persistence.

Trigeminal: The trigeminal nerve is the fifth cranial nerve, with three branches (ophthalmic, maxillary and mandibular), and is the principal sensory nerve of the face. The trigeminal component of olfaction is the sensation of hot, cold, tingling or irritation; for example, menthol has a smell that is perceived as 'cooling'.

Urinous: A term that describes an odour that resembles urine.

Volatile: Descriptive of a substance which evaporates when exposed to air. The term also applies to the low boiling-point constituents of natural aromatic materials; for example, plant volatile oils.

Volatility: The rate at which a substance evaporates. The concept of volatility has led to the classification of essential oils and aromatic extracts as top, middle and base notes.

REFERENCES

Aftel, M. (2008) *Essence and Alchemy: A Natural History of Perfume*. Layton, UT: Gibbs Smith.

Bahar-Fuchs, A., Moss, S., Rowe, C. and Savage, G. (2011) 'Awareness of olfactory deficits in healthy aging, amnestic mild cognitive impairment and Alzheimer's disease.' *International Psychogeriatrics 23*, 7, 1097–1106.

Barkat, S., Le Berre, E., Coureaud, G., Sicard, G. and Thomas-Danguin, T. (2012) 'Perceptual blending in odor mixtures depends on the nature of odorants and human olfactory expertise.' *Chemical Senses 37*, 159–166.

Bitter, T., Brüderle, J., Gudziol, H., Burmeister, H.P., Gaser, C. and Guntinas-Lichius, O. (2010) 'Gray and white matter reduction in hyposmic subjects : A voxel-based morphometry study.' *Brain Research 1347*, 42–47. Available at www.elsevier.com/locate/brainres, accessed on 7 March 2012.

Bloom, W. (2011) *The Power of Modern Spirituality*. London: Piatkus.

Burr, C. (2007) *The Perfect Scent*. New York, NY: Picador.

Butte College (date unknown) *Reasoning*. Available at www.butte.edu/departments/cas/tipsheets/thinking/reasoning.html, accessed on 5 November 2013.

Calkin, R.R. and Jellinek, J.S. (1994) *Perfumery: Practice and Principles*. New York, NY: John Wiley and Sons.

Carter, R. (2010) *Mapping the Mind*. London: Phoenix.

Curtis, T. and Williams, D.G. (2009) *Introduction to Perfumery*. Weymouth: Micelle Press.

Dalton, P. (1996) 'Cognitive aspects of perfumery.' *Perfumer & Flavorist 21*, 13–20.

Dalton, P. and Wysocki, C.J. (1996) 'The nature and duration of adaptation following long-term exposure to odors.' *Perception & Psychophysics 58*, 781–792. Cited in P. Dalton (1996) 'Cognitive aspects of perfumery.' *Perfumer & Flavorist 21*, 13–20.

Damholdt, M.F., Borghammer, P., Larsen, L. and Østergaard, K. (2011) 'Odor identification deficits identify Parkinson's disease patients with poor cognitive performance.' *Movement Disorders 21*, 11, 2045–2050.

Doty, R.L. (2009) 'Symposium overview: Do environmental agents enter the brain via the olfactory mucosa to induce neurodegenerative diseases?' *International Symposium on Olfaction and Taste 1170*, 610–614.

Erligmann, A. (2001) 'Sandalwood oils.' *International Journal of Aromatherapy 11*, 4, 186–192.

Fujii, N., Abla, D., Kudo, N., Hihara, S., Okanoya, K. and Iriki, A. (2007) 'Prefrontal activity during koh-do incense discrimination.' *Neuroscience Research 59*, 257–264.

Genter, M.B., Kendig, E.L. and Knutson, M.D. (2009) 'Uptake of materials from the nasal cavity into the blood and brain: Are we finally beginning to understand these processes at the molecular level?' *International Symposium on Olfaction and Taste 1170*, 623–628.

Hawkes, C.H. and Doty, R.L. (2009) *Neurology of Olfaction*. New York, NY: Cambridge University Press.

Hawkes, C.H., Tredici, K.D. and Braak, H. (2009) 'Parkinson's disease: The dual hit theory revisited.' *International Symposium on Olfaction and Taste 1170*, 615–622.

Huizinga, J. (1955) *Homo Ludens*. Boston: Beacon Press. Cited in K. Morita (1992) *The Book of Incense: Enjoying the Traditional Art of Japanese Scents*. Tokyo: Kodansha International.

Laska, M. and Ringh, A. (2010) 'How big is the gap between olfactory detection and recognition of aliphatic aldehydes?' *Attention, Perception & Psychophysics 72*, 3, 806–812.

Lawless, A. (2009) *Artisan Perfumery or Being Led by the Nose*. Stroud: Boronia Souk.

Lawless, A. (2010) *The Ordinary Mind, Perfume and Natural Health*. Available at at www.aleclawless.blogspot.co.uk, accessed on 21 June 2012.

Lawless, J. (2012) *The Encyclopedia of Essential Oils: The Complete Guide to the Use of Aromatic Oils in Aromatherapy, Herbalism, Health and Wellbeing*. London: Thorsons Publishing Group Ltd.

Livermore, A. and Laing, D.G. (1996) 'Influence of training and experience on the perception of multicomponent odor mixtures.' *Journal of Experimental Psychology, Human Perception and Performance 22*, 267–277.

Lombion-Pouthier, S., Vandel, P., Nezelhof, S., Haffen, E. and Millot, J.-L. (2006) 'Odor perception in patients with mood disorders.' *Journal of Affective Disorders 90*, 187–191.

Malaspina, D., Corcoran, C. and Goudsmit, N., (2006) Chapter 12: 'The impact of olfaction on human social functioning.' In W. Brewer, D. Castle and C. Pantelis (eds) *Olfaction and the Brain*. New York, NY: Cambridge University Press.

Morely, J.F., Weintraub, D., Mamikonyan, E., Moberg, P.J., Siderowf, A.D. and Duda, J.E. (2011) 'Olfactory dysfunction is associated with neuropsychiatric manifestations in Parkinson's disease.' *Movement Disorders 26*, 11, 2051–2057.

Morita, K. (1992) *The Book of Incense: Enjoying the Traditional Art of Japanese Scents*. Tokyo: Kodansha International.

Prediger, R.D.S., Rial, D., Medeiros, R., Figueiredo, C.P., Doty, R.L. and Takahashi, R.N. (2009) 'Disease.' *International Symposium on Olfaction and Taste 1170*, 629–636.

Quinn, A. (2012) 'A systematic literature review of attars: The history of emotional/physical uses with a view to present day applications within aromatherapy practices.' Dissertation. Edinburgh Napier University.

Rabin, M.D. and Cain, W.S. (1986) 'Determinants of measured olfactory sensitivity.' *Perception & Psychophysics 39*, 281–286. Cited in P. Dalton (1996) 'Cognitive aspects of perfumery.' *Perfumer & Flavorist 21*, 13–20.

Roudnitska, E. (1991) 'The Art of Perfumery.' In P.M. Müller and D. Lamparsky (eds) *Perfumes: Art, Science and Technology*. London: Elsevier. Cited in M. Aftel (2008) *Essence and Alchemy: A Natural History of Perfume*. Layton, UT: Gibbs Smith.

Semb, G. (1968) 'The detectability of the odor of butanol.' *Perception & Psychophysics 4*, 335–340. Cited in P. Dalton (1996) 'Cognitive aspects of perfumery.' *Perfumer & Flavorist 21*, 13–20.

Stansfield, W.D. (2012) 'Science and the senses: Perceptions and deceptions.' *The American Biology Teacher 74*, 145–150.

Tisserand, R. and Young, R. (2014) *Essential Oil Safety, 2nd Edition*. Edinburgh: Churchill Livingstone.

Tonutti, I. and Liddle, P. (2010) 'Aromatic plants in alcoholic beverages: A review.' *Flavour and Fragrance Journal 25*, 341–350.

Tsunetsugu, Y., Park, B.-J. and Miyazaki, Y. (2010) 'Trends in research related to "Shinrin-yoku" (taking in the forest atmosphere or forest bathing) in Japan.' *Environmental Health Preventative Medicine 15*, 27–37.

Turin, L. and Sanchez, T. (2009) *Perfumes: The A–Z Guide*. London: Profile Books.

Williams, D.G. (1995) *Odours: Their Description and Classification Part 1 Diploma Perfumery Correspondence Course*. London: Perfumery Education Centre.

Williams, D.G. (1996) *The Chemistry of Essential Oils*. Dorset: Micelle Press.

Williams, D.G. (2000) *Lecture Notes on Essential Oils*. Peterborough: Eve Taylor.

Zarzo, M. and Stanton, D.T. (2009) 'Understanding the underlying dimensions in perfumers' odor perception space as a basis for developing meaningful odor maps.' *Attention, Perception and Psychophysics 71*, 225–247.

Bibliography for olfactory profiles

Bowles, E.J. (2003) *The Chemistry of Aromatherapeutic Oils. (Third edition.)* Crows Nest: Allen and Unwin.

Burfield, T. (2002) 'Cedarwood oils.' *The Cropwatch Series*. Available at www.cropwatch. org, accessed on 31 November 2011.

Calkin, R.R. (2013) *The Fragrance of Old Roses*. Available at www.historicroses.org/index. php?id=38, accessed on 11 February 2013. (First published in the *Historic Rose Journal*, Spring 1999, No. 17.)

Curtis, T. and Williams, D.G. (2009) *Introduction to Perfumery*. Dorset: Micelle Press.

Erligmann, A. (2001) 'Sandalwood oils.' *International Journal of Aromatherapy 11*, 4, 186–192.

Gimelli, S.P. (2001) *Aroma Science*. Dorset: Micelle Press.

Jouhar, A.J. (ed.) (1991) *Poucher's Perfumes, Cosmetics and Soaps Volume 1: The Raw Materials of Perfumery. (Ninth edition.)* London: Chapman and Hall.

Lawless, A. (2009) *Artisan Perfumery or Being Led by the Nose*. Stroud: Boronia Souk.

Valder, C., Neugbauer, M., Meier, M. and Kohlenberg, B. (2003) 'Western Australian sandalwood oil: New constituents of Santalum spicatum (R.Br.) A. DC. (Santalaceae).' *Journal of Essential Oil Research*, May/June

Weyerstahl, P., Marschall, H., Weirauch, M., Thefeld, K. and Surburg, H. (1998) 'Constituents of commercial labdanum oil.' *Flavour and Fragrance Journal 13*, 295–318.

Williams, D.G. (1995a) *Odours: Their Description and Classification Part 1 Diploma Perfumery Correspondence Course*. London: Perfumery Education Centre.

Williams, D.G. (1995b) *Aromatic Materials from Natural Sources Part 2 Diploma Perfumery Correspondence Course*. London: Perfumery Education Centre.

Williams, D.G. (1996) *The Chemistry of Essential Oils*. Dorset: Micelle Press.

Williams, D.G. (2000) *Lecture Notes on Essential Oils*. Peterborough: Eve Taylor.

SOME SUPPLIERS OF AROMATIC MATERIALS

UK
Aqua Oleum
www.aqua-oleum.co.uk

Ellwoods of Dumfries
www.ellwoodsofdumfries.co.uk

Neat Wholesale
www.neatwholesale.co.uk

Oshadi UK
www.oshadhi.co.uk

Quinessence
www.quinessence.co.uk

USA
Eden Botanicals
www.edenbotanicals.com

Oshadi USA
www.oshadhiusa.com

Snow Lotus Inc.
www.snowlotus.org

White Lotus Aromatics
www.whitelotusaromatics.com

Europe
Albert Vieille (France)
www.albertvieille.com

Biolandes (France)
www.biolandes.com

Néroliane (France)
www.neroliane.fr

La Via del Profumo (Italy)
www.profumo.it

Australia
Sydney Essential Oil co.
www.seoc.com.au

Education
The Perfumery Art School
www.perfumeartschool-uk.com

The Perfume Foundation
www.perfumefoundation.org

SCENT INDEX

SUBJECT INDEX

AUTHOR INDEX

ABOUT THE AUTHOR

Jennifer Peace Rhind is a Chartered Biologist with a PhD in Mycotoxicology from the University of Strathclyde. Her long-standing interest in Complementary and Alternative Medicine (CAM) has led to qualifications in massage and aromatherapy, and for 13 years she worked as a therapist and partner in a multidisciplinary complementary healthcare clinic. During this time she became involved in CAM education in the private sector and co-founded the first professionally accredited CAM school in Scotland. She was a lecturer in Complementary Healthcare at Edinburgh Napier University for 14 years, and remains involved in scent education. Jennifer is the author of *Essential Oils, Fragrance and Wellbeing* and *A Sensory Journey*, all published by Singing Dragon. She lives in Biggar near the Scottish Borders.